Bereavement Care:
A New Look at Hospice and Community Based Services

Bereavement Care:
A New Look at Hospice and Community Based Services

Marcia E. Lattanzi-Licht
Jane Marie Kirschling
Stephen Fleming
Editors

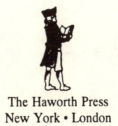

The Haworth Press
New York • London

Bereavement Care: A New Look at Hospice and Community Based Services has also been published as *The Hospice Journal*, Volume 5, Number 1 1989.

The Haworth Press, Inc., 10 Alice Street, Binghamton, NY 13904-1580
EUROSPAN/Haworth, 3 Henrietta Street, London WC2E 8LU England

Library of Congress Cataloging-in-Publication Data

Bereavement care : a new look at hospice and community based services / Marcia E. Lattanzi-Licht, Jane Marie Kirschling, Stephen Fleming, editors.
    p. cm.
  Bibliography: p.
  ISBN 0-86656-944-8
  1. Bereavement—Psychological aspects. 2. Hospice care. I. Lattanzi-Licht, Marcia E. II. Kirschling, Jane Marie. III. Fleming, Stephen (Stephen J.)
RC455.4.L67B47   1989
155.9′37—dc20   89-11038
                                                     CIP

Bereavement Care: A New Look at Hospice and Community Based Services

CONTENTS

ABOUT THE EDITORS

Marcia E. Lattanzi-Licht, RN, MA, is a consultant, educator and psychotherapist. An internationally known speaker, she has appeared on the Today Show and numerous other television and radio programs. Currently, she maintains a private psychotherapy practice in Boulder, Colorado, and works as a consultant with numerous hospitals, law enforcement agencies, local and county governments, home care and hospice programs and other professional groups locally and across North America. She was a founder of Boulder County Hospice, Colorado, and the originator and director of its nationally recognized education and bereavement programs.

Jane Marie Kirschling, RN, DNS, is Associate Professor, Department of Family Nursing, School of Nursing, The Oregon Health Sciences University, Portland, Oregon. For years, she worked for various hospice organizations as a nurse, providing direct care for the terminally ill and their families. Dr. Kirschling is currently Co-Chair of the Bereavement Network, Portland, Oregon, a community based group for persons who work with the bereaved. She has published and presented widely on the topics of bereavement, social support, and hospice care.

Stephen J. Fleming, PhD, is Associate Professor, Department of Psychology, Atkinson College, York University, Ontario, Canada. He is also in private practice in Brampton, Ontario. An editorial board member of the *Journal of Palliative Care*, Dr. Fleming has published extensively and spoken internationally in the area of dying and bereavement.

Preface

The story of any one man's real experience finds its starting
parallel in that of every one of us.

James Russel Lowell

While bereavement care is an important value and a differentiating characteristic to hospices, it has received scattered attention and
the allocation of often minimal resources. Seen as an add-on or less
than essential service, bereavement programs struggle for clarity,
quality and consistency.

The papers in this collection provide an interdisciplinary look at
some key bereavement care concerns. We have often stumbled over
what hospice bereavement care entails, as each program sets individual goals and approaches. In this collection there is some attempt
to look at the structure and function of Hospice Bereavement Programs, from research that examines services provided and providers, to clinical articles that explore the role of the volunteer and a
model of group services. In addition there is a look at grief assessment and the evaluation of various tools.

Because often, as Goethe says, "we see what we know," this
special edition attempts to broaden our understanding of grief by
presenting some new attempts to look at theories and frameworks.
The material in this collection covers a broad spectrum of topics,
interests and perspectives from divergent disciplines and clinical
experiences. Jane Kirschling, Stephen Fleming and I solicited a
range of articles from a variety of persons who we felt would have a
valuable contribution to make to this exploration of Hospice Bereavement Services. We were not always in agreement with the
material presented by the contributing authors, but attempted to include a range of voices that would also challenge and stimulate
future work. The involvement of this editorial team, representing a

ix

mix of disciplines and perspectives, was valuable to the shaping of this diverse offering.

Perhaps this volume raises more questions than it addresses. Our goal was to contribute to the exploration and examination of concerns that could be strong influencing factors in the quality of Hospice Bereavement Services. We encourage all those involved in these services to continue the work of defining, refining and evaluating this important and symbolic area of hospice care.

Finally, Jane Kirschling and Stephen Fleming deserve my thanks for so generously devoting their considerable energy and skills to this effort. Their involvement made this collection richer, and a truly broad-based look at bereavement care.

Marcia E. Lattanzi-Licht

Bereavement Services: Practice and Problems

Marcia E. Lattanzi-Licht

SUMMARY. Hospice bereavement services vary widely and are often loosely defined. This paper describes the results of a survey on the form and function of hospice bereavement services completed by NHO Provider Member hospices. It explores issues related to staffing, training, size, services provided, and service priorities. Additionally, data collection and research, referrals, funding, risk assessment, obstacles programs face and the limitations that are inherent in hospice structures are examined. These important elements are presented along with a discussion of critical issues and recommendations for future research and study.

Historically, hospices have placed a high value on the provision of family-centered care, and support to family members following the death of their loved one. In fact, this identifying characteristic of a hospice has become a factor which differentiates hospices from other home care or inpatient programs. Yet, bereavement services

Marcia E. Lattanzi-Licht, RN, MA, is affiliated with Comprehensive Psychological Services Group. She is a clinician and lecturer in the areas of loss, professional stress, team building and conflict management. A founder of Boulder County Hospice, she was the originator and director of its Bereavement and Education programs for nine years. Currently a consultant and psychotherapist in private practice, she continues to lecture internationally. She also has worked extensively with law enforcement and first responder groups and as a management trainer/consultant for the National Academy of Correction.

The author would like to express her appreciation to Martin Schaefer and the administrative staff of Boulder County Hospice for their help with the initial research project.

Address correspondence to the author at Comprehensive Psychological Services Group, 1526 Spruce St., Suite 301, Boulder, CO 80302.

1

in hospices suffer under the weight of some unique developmental and practical problems.

Bereavement programs have often been formally developed after other hospice services have been provided for a period of time. With the passage of the Hospice Medicare legislation in 1982, the exclusion of reimbursement for bereavement services was rooted in some of the same concerns about the unclear nature and undocumented effectiveness of bereavement services that still trouble hospices today.

In the passage of the hospice legislation, some legislators reacted to bereavement support as the realm of one's personal clergy, not of a hospice, and pressed for exclusion of this service from the bill. Also, at the time of the proposed Medicare legislation, there was little documentation of hospice bereavement services, or of their effectiveness. In contrast to the more definable nature of other hospice services, bereavement support was a vague catch-all term that included such diverse activities as continuing phone calls from the hospice nurse, hospice memorial service rituals, visits by a social worker or a bereavement volunteer, and correspondence or support groups.

Another part of the difficulty with bereavement services rests in the "poor stepchild" view hospices now take of them. The legislative disincentive to the provision of hospice bereavement support at the time when all hospice services were developing and evolving has clearly influenced and limited today's "state of the art" in bereavement care. Because bereavement services are largely preventive and palliative services, they parallel the lower priority ranking of preventive services in mental health settings.

This article will explore the form and function of today's hospice bereavement services. The author was unable to find any similar projects in a search of the literature, and is unaware of any other efforts to examine the current functioning and makeup of hospice bereavement services. Relevant references are integrated throughout the body of the paper.

This article reports the results of the Bereavement Services Survey project, and will then discuss their implications and relevance to hospice bereavement services. The survey described here has also subsequently been adapted and administered by Glennie and completed by members of the Colorado Hospice Organization. A description of those results and clinical comments by Ann Luke are forthcoming.

METHOD

The author's experience in developing and directing the Bereavement Program at Boulder County Hospice (1977-1985) led to a continuing interest in bereavement care and in the broad nature and ambiguity of hospice bereavement services. In late 1986, as a private practitioner, the author collaborated with Boulder County Hospice in the mailing of a 2-page, 21-item "Bereavement Services Survey" to 439 Provider Members of the National Hospice Organization. Provider Member status is a membership designation that is part of the dues structure that implies active delivery of hospice services and confers NHO voting privileges.

The questionnaire requested that respondents fill in the blanks, check items, and complete four open-ended questions. An introductory letter was included with the questionnaire informing respondents that the information would be used in a presentation by the author at a pre-conference seminar of the National Hospice Organization's Annual Meeting in Denver in November 1986. There was also a commitment to publish the findings in either *The Hospice Journal* or the *NHO Hospice Team Quarterly*. The letter from the author and the survey were addressed to the "Bereavement Services Coordinator," and a self-addressed, unstamped envelope was included. There was a 61% return (N = 268) of the questionnaires.

RESULTS

Development of Bereavement Services

A composite look at 266 of the responding hospice programs indicated that the hospices ranged in age from a "new" program, or programs just beginning the delivery of services to those providing services for 11 years and 2 months. The average age of the responding hospices was 5.3 years.

Responses (n = 253) to the question of how long the hospice

TABLE 1

BEREAVEMENT SERVICES SURVEY

NHO PROVIDER MEMBERS	N=439
RESPONSES	N=268
PERCENT OF TOTAL SAMPLE	61%

HOSPICE SIZE

AVERAGE DEATHS PER YEAR	92
RANGE	10-900

---

program had been delivering bereavement services indicated a range of "new" services, or services just being initiated at the time of completion of the questionnaire to the provision of services for 10 years. The average age for bereavement service programs was 4.5 years, a 9-month differential from the onset of the hospice program of care. This difference could be related to the practical development or evolution of "after care" services subsequent to the provision of services to care for the dying. However, it is important to note that a few of the hospices, particularly those in some rural or tourist areas, began their hospice programs with the provision of community-wide bereavement services, including services in situations of sudden, accidental deaths.

Size Factors

Of the hospices responding to the survey, 255 reported an average of 92 deaths per year in their programs. The range included 10 to 900 deaths per year. As will be discussed later, the element of size and the number of deaths per year seem to be major influences upon the type of bereavement services offered by a hospice program.

Coordination of Services

One of the dimensions that the Hospice Bereavement Services survey explored was that of leadership or coordination of care. In asking the title of the person coordinating bereavement services, of a total 201 responses, 97 programs (48%) indicated that the most frequently used title was "Bereavement Coordinator." Other title forms included in this category were "Director of Bereavement," "Coordinator of After Care" and "Family Support Coordinator."

In a number of hospices (n = 28, 14%), particularly the smaller hospice programs, the coordination of bereavement services was the responsibility of the Hospice Coordinator or the Hospice Director. In 19 programs (9%), the title "Social Worker" was listed for the coordinator of bereavement services, while in 15 programs (7.5%) the "Director of Social Services" was listed. Together these represent 17.0% (n = 34) of the respondents. A number of programs (n = 17, 8.5%) listed the Volunteer Coordinator as the person responsible for bereavement services. Other disciplines listed as the titled coordinators of bereavement services include the "Chaplain" (n = 9, 4.5%), the "Patient Care Coordinator" (n = 7, 3.5%), and the "Bereavement Counselor" (n = 7, 3.5%).

A significant number of programs (n = 49, 24%) listed dual roles under the "title" of the individual coordinating bereavement services. The "Director of Volunteers and Bereavement" was responsible for coordination in 8.5% of the hospices surveyed (n = 17). In 7 hospices (3.5%) the Volunteer Coordinator and the Social Worker jointly coordinated bereavement services, while 4 programs (2%) cited both the Social Worker and Bereavement Coordinator. It is assumed that in these programs the Social Worker's role would be one of clinical supervision.

A small number of programs cited the joining of roles of the Volunteer Coordinator and Chaplain, of the Bereavement Coordinator and the Hospice Nurse, and the efforts of Hospice Nurses and Volunteers as a group in the coordination of bereavement services. Bereavement services are a shared responsibility coordinated by a group of two or more persons, such as "Co-Directors" and a "Be-

TABLE 2

COORDINATION OF BEREAVEMENT SERVICES

TOTAL RESPONSES = 201

TITLE	NUMBER	PERCENT [a]
BEREAVEMENT COORDINATOR	97	48.0
SOCIAL WORKER/DIRECTOR OF SOCIAL SERVICES	34	17.0
HOSPICE DIRECTOR	28	14.0
VOLUNTEER COORDINATOR	17	8.5
CHAPLAIN	9	4.5
PATIENT CARE COORDINATOR	7	3.5
BEREAVEMENT COUNSELOR	7	3.5
OTHER	2	1.0
DUAL ROLES		
DIRECTOR OF VOLUNTEERS AND BEREAVEMENT	17	8.5
DIRECTOR OF VOLUNTEERS AND SOCIAL WORK	7	3.5
SOCIAL WORK AND BEREAVEMENT COORDINATOR	4	2.0
BEREAVEMENT COMMITTEE	4	2.0

a   Percentages are rounded to the nearest .5%

reavement Committee'' in 2% (n = 4) of the responding hospice programs.

Discipline of Coordinator

In a separate listing, respondents were asked to identify the discipline of the individual coordinating bereavement services. Of 212 responses, Social Work represented 36% (n = 76) and Nursing represented 24.5% (n = 52) of the responses. The ''Social Work'' discipline listing included Master's and Bachelor level persons, as well as ''Sociology'' and ''Social Services'' designations. Various levels of nursing education were included in its discipline listing, including Registered Nurses, Bachelor and Master's level educated, and other discipline advanced degrees coupled with nursing, such as a Master of Arts or a Master of Public Health.

''Clergy'' or ''Pastoral Counselors,'' including Master of Divinity levels of education were indicated by 11.5% of the programs (n = 24). In 10% (n = 21) of the hospices, ''Counseling'' was listed as the discipline coordinating bereavement services, and included Master's-prepared persons. ''Psychology'' was cited by 3% (n = 7) of those responding, while 8.5% of the persons coordinating bereavement services represented mixed disciplines (n = 18). The remaining hospices noted that their bereavement programs were led by other disciplines including lay or hospice-trained persons (n = 7, 3%), or by persons with a background in ''Education'' (n = 5, 2.5%), ''Occupational Therapy,'' or ''Human Development and Family Studies.''

Salaried and Volunteer Coordination

Another aspect of the coordination of bereavement services involves whether the coordinator functions as a salaried staff member or as a volunteer. This information was coupled with the number of hours worked per week on the coordination of bereavement services. The vast majority of total respondents (N = 260) were salaried at some level (N = 221, 85%). An average of 11.5 salaried hours were spent weekly on the coordination of bereavement services. A number of coordinators (n = 28, 11%) listed that they

TABLE 3

DISCIPLINE OF COORDINATOR

TOTAL RESPONSES = 212

	NUMBER	PERCENT	
SOCIAL WORK	76	36.0	a
NURSING	52	24.5	
CLERGY	24	11.5	
COUNSELING	21	10.0	
MIXED DISCIPLINES (2 OR MORE)	18	8.5	
PSYCHOLOGY	7	3.0	
LAY PERSONS	7	3.0	
EDUCATION	5	2.5	
OTHER	2	1.0	

---

a   Percentages are rounded to the nearest .5%

spent both salaried and volunteer hours on coordination on a weekly basis. Volunteer hours spent on bereavement coordination averaged just under 10 hours per week. For programs where coordination was solely a volunteer activity (n = 37, 14%), an average of 8 hours was spent per week on coordination.

Bereavement Personnel

Respondents to the Bereavement Services Survey were asked to fill in numbers of staff, volunteers and students offering formal bereavement follow-up services. Differences in programs, and in program design created a range of responses. A number of hospices indicated that they had no specific bereavement personnel, or that all personnel were involved in follow-up of families. One response noted that the 11 staff listed as involved in follow-up included the nurses, who were responsible for the bereavement assessment.

Several programs seemed to list all hospice volunteers, and one indicated that "all 80 volunteers can be assigned to bereavement follow-up when appropriate." Another respondent indicated that none offer "formal" bereavement follow-up services. Several respondents were not clear on the definition of "formal bereavement follow-up services." The author saw "formal" bereavement ser-

TABLE 4

SALARIED AND VOLUNTEER COORDINATION

TOTAL RESPONSES = 260

	NUMBER	PERCENT
SALARIED AT SOME LEVEL	221	85.0 [a]
SALARIED AND VOLUNTEER HOURS SPENT ON WEEKLY COORDINATION	28	11.0
VOLUNTEER ONLY ACTIVITY	37	14.0

	HOURS/WEEK
AVERAGE SALARIED HOURS FOR BEREAVEMENT COORDINATION	11.5
AVERAGE VOLUNTEER HOURS FOR BEREAVEMENT COORDINATION	10
AVERAGE HOURS FOR BEREAVEMENT COORDINATION AS VOLUNTEER ONLY	8

[a]   PERCENTAGES ARE ROUNDED TO THE NEAREST .5%

9

vices as those of a standardized design, and administered by specific persons under the supervision of a named and qualified staff person. Informal services include random phone calls or visits that are at the discretion and convenience of staff or volunteers involved with the family prior to the death.

Of the 200 responses about the number of staff involved in formal follow-up, a total of 728 persons were indicated, an average of 3.6 staff persons per program. Hospices showed a total of 2774 volunteers involved in follow-up in 186 programs for an average of almost 15 volunteers per hospice. However, only 28 responding hospices utilized a total of 49 students, at an average of 1.8 students in each of those programs. Table 5 lists the ranges in the numbers of staff, volunteers and students involved in formal bereavement follow-up.

Bereavement Staff Training

While training is a standard of hospice programs of care, there is little uniformity of training programs or content. The Bereavement Services Survey contained a question about whether the bereavement staff received initial training, and if so, the number of hours of the training. Of a total 256 responses, 237 programs (92.5%) showed that they offered initial training for bereavement staff. The average number of hours spent on this initial training was 16 (range 2-40). Although the question asked if bereavement staff receives initial training, most of the responses seemed to indicate or give reference to the general hospice training program. The questionnaire did not ask respondents whether this training was the same initial training offered to all program volunteers or staff.

In the comments made by respondents, 24 (9.5%) listed specific numbers of hours in addition to the general hospice training. These additional or specialized bereavement training hours averaged 8 per program. Also, 11 hospices (4.5%) showed that they offered ongoing training and continuing education for their bereavement staff, including inservices, seminars, workshops and periodic support meetings.

Hospices that did not offer initial training for their bereavement staff totaled 19 (7.5%). These programs cited the fact that only

TABLE 5

BEREAVEMENT PERSONNEL

STAFF

TOTAL RESPONSES = 200

TOTAL NUMBER OF STAFF INVOLVED
IN FORMAL BEREAVEMENT CARE   728
AVERAGE STAFF PER PROGRAM
IN FORMAL BEREAVEMENT CARE   3.6

VOLUNTEERS

TOTAL RESPONSES =186

TOTAL NUMBER OF VOLUNTEERS INVOLVED   2774
IN FORMAL BEREAVEMENT CARE
AVERAGE VOLUNTEERS PER PROGRAM
IN FORMAL BEREAVEMENT CARE   15

STUDENTS

TOTAL RESPONSES = 28

TOTAL NUMBER OF STUDENTS INVOLVED
IN FORMAL BEREAVEMENT CARE   49
AVERAGE STUDENTS PER UTILIZING
PROGRAM IN BEREAVMENT CARE   1.8

professionals or staff members, not volunteers, handled bereavement follow-up.

Services Provided

An important question in the delivery of bereavement care and services centers around who should receive follow-up. Hospices responding to the Bereavement Services Survey were asked to estimate the percentage of bereaved persons who receive personal bereavement contacts after the death of their loved one (i.e., phone

TABLE 6

BEREAVEMENT STAFF TRAINING

TOTAL RESPONSES = 256

	NUMBER	PERCENT
OFFER INITIAL TRAINING	237	92.5 a
AVERAGE HOURS OF INITIAL TRAINING = 16		
RANGE OF HOURS = 2 - 40		
ADDITIONAL BEREAVEMENT TRAINING HOURS	24	9.5
AVERAGE ADDITIONAL HOURS = 8		
ONGOING TRAINING	11	4.5
DID NOT OFFER TRAINING	19	7.5

---

a   Percentages are rounded to the nearest .5%

calls, visits, group sessions). Estimates by the 258 responders were that over 89% of bereaved family members received personal contacts (range = 10%-100%).

Another question asked respondents to check the bereavement services that their hospices provided. Of the 11 services specifically listed, 266 hospices giving multiple responses estimated that "phone calls by bereavement personnel" was the most commonly offered service (n = 235, 88.5%). Almost 83% of the hospices (n = 221) provide the follow-up service of "phone calls by the nurse involved prior to the death." The third most frequently offered service was "visits to the bereaved by bereavement personnel" (n = 220, 83%). Other frequently offered services were "letters or notices to the bereaved regarding meetings or group offerings" and "literature and materials on grief" (n = 217, 81.5%). "Visits to the bereaved by the nurse" ranked as another prevalent service at 74% (n = 196), while 70% of the programs offered "group meetings" (n = 186). Over 64.5% of hospices (n = 171) offer "memorial services" to bereaved family members, and 56.5% (n = 150) showed "correspondence on grief sent to the bereaved." "Courses or group series" are offered by almost 38% of the programs, but only 14.5% (n = 39) offer a "newsletter for the bereaved." Only a small number of programs filled in the "other" blank category to indicate that they offer "individual counseling," "social offerings," "seasonal cards," and a "men's group."

Service Priorities

From the listing of the services discussed, and shown in Table 7, or adding their own, respondents were asked to list the actual or functional priority of bereavement services delivered in their hospice, filling in the first, second and third priorities. "Visits to the bereaved" was listed as the "first priority" by 110 programs, or 47%. The "second priority" was "phone calls to the bereaved," indicated by 56 hospices, or 24% of responders. Additionally, 56 programs (24%) listed "phone calls to the bereaved" as their "first priority." "Group meetings" was the most frequent "third priority" with 50 programs, or 21.5% of the responders. All other services listed for any of the priority ranking positions totaled less than 12%.

Referrals

Because hospice programs generally identify that their scope of care involves support around the normal grief response, the survey asked NHO Provider Member Hospices to estimate what percentage of their bereavement clients would seek, or be referred to outside counseling. With a range of .5% to 30%, 240 hospices estimated that an average of 6.5% of their clients sought or were referred to outside counseling.

Risk Assessment

The National Academy of Science, Institute of Medicine publication, *Bereavement: Reactions, Consequences and Care* (Osterweis et al., 1984) posits that the lack of ability to define outcomes and criteria for adequate recovery makes it difficult to identify and measure risk factors. And yet, one of the goals and standards of hospice bereavement care that is formally acknowledged by the National Hospice Organization's Hospice Standards of Care (1980), the Medicare interpretive guidelines, the Joint Commission on the Ac-

TABLE 7

SERVICES PROVIDED

TOTAL RESPONSES = 258

ESTIMATED % OF BEREAVED PERSONS
RECEIVING PERSONAL BEREAVEMENT CONTACTS = 89%
RANGE = .10 -100%

SPECIFIC SERVICES

RESPONSES = 266 (BASED ON MULTIPLE RESPONSES)

	NUMBER	PERCENT
	235	88.5 a
PHONE CALLS BY BEREAVEMENT PERSONNEL	221	83.0
PHONE CALLS BY RN INVOLVED PRIOR TO DEATH	220	83.0
VISITS BY BEREAVEMENT PERSONNEL	217	81.5
LETTERS/NOTICES OF GROUPS/MEETINGS	217	81.5
LITERATURE/MATERIALS ON GRIEF	196	74.0
VISITS BY RN INVOLVED PRIOR TO DEATH	186	70.0
GROUP MEETINGS	171	64.5
MEMORIAL SERVICES	150	56.5
CORRESPONDANCE ON GRIEF SENT	101	38.0
COURSES OR GROUP SERIES	39	14.5
BEREAVEMENT NEWSLETTER SENT	10	4.0
OTHER: INDIVIDUAL COUNSELING	3	1.0
SOCIAL EVENTS		

a   PERCENTAGES ROUNDED TO THE NEAREST .5%

TABLE 8

REFERRALS TO OUTSIDE COUNSELING

TOTAL RESPONSES = 210
AVERAGE = 6.5%
RANGE = .05 - 30%

---

creditation of Hospitals requirements and the literature on bereavement involves the assessment of "High Risk Factors" (Lattanzi, 1979; Parkes, 1981; O'Toole, 1985). In the Bereavement Services Survey, hospices were asked whether they currently used any bereavement assessment process for identifying "high risk" individuals, and if so, what type. Of 265 hospice program responses, 77% (n = 204) reported the use of a bereavement assessment process for identifying "high risk" individuals. Of those, 57.5% (n = 118) described the "type" of assessment used as a written "form" that their hospice had developed. A number of programs specifically indicated the use of Parkes' "Risk Assessment" Scale (n = 16, 8%), while others (n = 11, 5.5%) cited the use of the American Medical Records Association "Bereavement Assessment" (Form #16, 1984), or the J.C.A.H. form. It is believed that others use these assessment tools, but did not name them directly.

Another group of programs (n = 61, 23%) indicated that they did not use any assessment process for identifying "high risk" individuals. It is speculated that this group would include the smaller, non-Medicare certified hospice programs. There was a wide range of responses to this question, with many of the hospices indicating that they have developed their own assessment tool/process. Often certain key staff members, i.e., social workers, or nurses were responsible for the formal assessment. A number of programs indicated that their assessment process was "informal," or a matter of discussion/judgement of the interdisciplinary team. A question that arose for the author involves the criteria that are used to measure or assess "high risk" bereaved persons.

TABLE 9

```
------------------------------------------------------------
                    HIGH RISK ASSESSMENT

TOTAL RESPONSES = 265
                                    NUMBER        PERCENT
YES                                   204           77.0
NO                                     61           23.0

------------------------------------------------------------
TYPE OF ASSESSMENT N=204
FORM OF OWN DESIGN                    118           57.5
PARKES                                16            8.0
AMRA/JCAH                             11            5.5
UNSPECIFIED                           59           29.0

```

Who Receives Services

Because of the individual nature of the bereavement programs in hospices, the survey questioned respondents about "which bereaved individuals receive services" in their program. Those completing the questionnaire were free to check multiple responses from the following list:

A. All
B. "High Risk" persons only
C. Personal contact with all
D. Personal contact with "High Risk" only
E. Written invitations to all
F. Other (please explain)

A total of 392 multiple responses showed that "personal contacts with all" was the most frequent designation (n = 129, 33%), closely followed by "written invitations to all" (n = 126, 32%). In 26.5% (n = 104) of the responding hospices, services were shown to be delivered to "all" bereaved individuals. There seems to be little inclination to provide "personal contact with 'high risk' only" (n = 13, 3%), or to support "'high risk' persons only" (n = 6, 1.5%). Responses offered in the "other" category included "telephone contact only" (n = 7, 2%), or "special attention to 'high risk' bereaved persons." Others indicated that the "family must request" bereavement services, or the services are provided "unless the family refuses," and also that services are "prioritized depending upon resources."

Obstacles

There is a distinct set of concerns surrounding bereavement programs as underdeveloped service components that include their lack of clear definition and the lack of research validation of any measurable "results" (de St. Aubin & Lund, 1986; Lattanzi, 1982, 1988; Osterweis et al., 1984). The Bereavement Services Survey asked each hospice to check the "greatest difficulties or obstacles encountered in the delivery of bereavement services" from the following list, with the option to check multiple items.

> A. Lack of organizational support of bereavement services
> B. Funding pressures
> C. Lack of sufficient staff time
> D. Lack of personnel
> E. Insufficient training
> F. Complexity/difficulty in defining bereavement services
> G. Staff or volunteer stress or burnout
> H. Other

The greatest obstacle to delivery of bereavement services shown by respondents was the "lack of sufficient staff time" (n = 206, 30%). There was a total of 694 responses to this particular item, the largest multiple response number in the survey. Secondly, the obstacle most frequently identified by respondents was the "lack of personnel" (n = 152, 22%). "Funding pressures" were cited as the third most significant obstacle by 14.5% (N = 101) of the multiple responses.

The obstacle that was termed "staff or volunteer burnout" was the fourth most frequently indicated obstacle at 10% (N = 70). Other obstacles noted were the "complexity/difficulty in defining

TABLE 10

SERVICES RECEIVED

TOTAL RESPONSES = 392 (BASED ON MULTIPLE RESPONSES)

	NUMBER	PERCENT	
ALL	104	26.5	a
"HIGH RISK" PERSONS ONLY	6	1.5	
PERSONAL CONTACT WITH ALL	129	33.0	
PERSONAL WITH "HIGH RISK" ONLY	13	3.0	
WRITTEN INVITATIONS TO ALL	126	32.0	
OTHER: TELEPHONE CONTACT ONLY	7	2.0	
OTHER	7	2.0	

a   Percentages are rounded to the nearest .5%

bereavement services'' (n = 61, 8.5%), and the "lack of organizational support" (n = 54, 8%). Only 5.5% (n = 40) indicated that "insufficient training" was an obstacle to the delivery of bereavement services. "Other" responses included the "person acknowledging the need," "distance" and "geographical area," "the lack of volunteer interest," or of "an organized bereavement service/team." While the indication of multiple obstacles diluted the individual percentages, the ranking was a clear indication and ordering of programmatic problems.

Program Funding

The value of services to an organization can often be correlated to the dollars allocated to them in the budgeting process. Another survey question examined the "amount budgeted this year for bereavement services," and the "percentage of the total annual budget" that it represented in the Provider Member Hospices. While a significant number of respondents noted that bereavement services were not specified or separated out in the hospice budget, an average of $13,014 was budgeted by 100 hospices with a range of responses of $50 to $90,000. The average of 87 hospices responding showed a 7% budget allotment for bereavement services with a range of .005 to 25%. Again, a number of hospices stated that bereavement services were not a budget item, or that the budget amount was unknown.

Data Collection and Research

With the belief that data collection and research are necessary elements in the continuation and development of hospice bereavement services, hospices surveyed were asked about their activities in these two areas. Of 252 responses, almost 40% were collecting

TABLE 11

BEREAVEMENT SERVICES: OBSTACLES

TOTAL RESPONSES = 694 (BASED ON MULTIPLE RESPONSES)

	NUMBER	PERCENT
LACK OF ORGANIZATIONAL SUPPORT	54	8.0
FUNDING PRESSURES	101	14.5
LACK OF STAFF TIME	206	30.0
LACK OF PERSONNEL	152	22.0
INSUFFICIENT TRAINING	40	5.5
COMPLEXITY/DIFFICULTY IN DEFINING BEREAVEMENT SERVICES	61	8.5
STAFF OR VOLUNTEER STRESS OR BURNOUT	70	10.0
OTHER	10	1.5

a   Percentages are rounded to the nearest .5%

TABLE 12

BEREAVEMENT PROGRAM FUNDING

AVERAGE AMOUNT BUDGETED   IOO RESPONSES = $13,014.
(RANGE = $50. - $90,000.)

AVERAGE PERCENTAGE OF TOTAL BUDGET   87 RESPONSES = 7%
(RANGE = .005% - 25%)

bereavement data, while over 60% (n = 152) reported that they were not currently collecting any bereavement data. The data that was explained or described in comments included the collection of statistics, demographic data and the completion of consumer surveys. Participation in research was an activity that only 15 of the 251 responding hospices reported (6%). The vast majority indicated that they were not engaged in any research activities (n = 236, 94%). Several explained that they had in the past cooperated with doctoral-level researchers, or that they had projects planned for the future.

Beyond Limitations

In the hope of acknowledging and stimulating possibilities, the survey questioned respondents about the "type of bereavement services they would offer if time and money were not limitations." Hospices filled in 396 multiple responses to this question. The most frequent response by hospice programs was that they would offer "more groups" (n = 122, 31%). Following significantly behind, hospices would like a "bereavement coordinator" or "more staff coordination" of their bereavement services (n = 62, 15.5%).

Hospices participating in the survey also showed that they would like to offer more "regular visits" (n = 49, 12%), or "more personal counseling" (n = 43, 11%). Additionally, 29 programs indicated that they would like to offer more "educational programs"

TABLE 13

DATA COLLECTION AND RESEARCH

TOTAL RESPONSES = 252 (BASED ON MULTIPLE RESPONSES)

	NUMBER	PERCENT
COLLECTING BEREAVEMENT DATA	100	40
NOT CURRENTLY COLLECTING BEREAVEMENT DATA	152	60

TOTAL RESPONSES = 251 (BASED ON MULTIPLE RESPONSES)

PARTICIPATING IN RESEARCH	15	6
NO RESEARCH ACTIVITIES	236	94

(7%), or have "additional resources" such as books, pamphlets, films, etc. (n = 23, 6%). "More mailings" were listed by 26 hospices (6.5%). Also, a number of programs (n = 26, 6.5%) stated that without the limitations of time and money, they would offer "probably the same" services. Finally, 13 programs (3.5%) indicated a desire for a "team of bereavement volunteers" while 2 wished to provide a "prevention program" while another would like to offer a "bereavement hot line."

DISCUSSION

Any attempt to problem-solve or plan for hospice bereavement services in the future must be based upon a realistic knowledge of their current status. This survey points out the wide range of services that fall under the umbrella of "hospice bereavement care." While this survey is a collection of significant information about the specific nature of hospice bereavement programs, it has limitations.

TABLE 14

BEYOND LIMITATIONS

IF TIME AND MONEY WERE NO OBJECT...

TOTAL RESPONSES = 396

	NUMBER	PERCENT	
MORE GROUPS	122	31.0	a
BEREAVEMENT COORDINATOR/ MORE STAFF COORDINATION	62	15.5	
MORE REGULAR VISITS	49	12.0	
MORE PERSONAL COUNSELING	43	11.0	
MORE EDUCATIONAL PROGRAMS	29	7.0	
MORE MAILINGS	26	6.5	
PROBABLY THE SAME	26	6.5	
ADDITIONAL RESOURCES (BOOKS, PAMPHLETS, FILMS)	23	6.0	
TEAM OF BEREAVEMENT VOLUNTEERS	13	3.5	
OTHER	3	1.0	

a   Percentages are rounded to the nearest .5%

Though the items were reviewed by a number of bereavement coordinators, and then revised, some of the questions were still not clear to respondents. The questions were generally directed toward information about formal services. The fact that all hospices consider that they offer bereavement services, whether formal programs or casual efforts, complicated the results. An additional problem arose from the lack of cross-referencing of materials as to program size. The Bereavement Services Survey did not differentiate or cross-reference age or size with the data gathered. These two factors would greatly color the delivery of services and the survey responses gathered. It would have been valuable to know the status of the program regarding Medicare certification and licensure. Also, since the items were self-report and self-estimate items in an area of service where there may be some feelings of failure to live up to personal standards, inflation of the responses is possible. Still, the large size of the total sample gives the data considerable weight.

Interest in Bereavement Services

One can conclude that there is considerable interest on the part of hospices in bereavement services. In addition to the significant number of surveys returned (n = 268, 61%), many respondents requested follow-up information. Also, numerous program coordinators attended the NHO Pre-Conference Seminar presented by the author in both 1986 and 1987 that incorporated this material. This parallels the findings of Simson and Wilson (1986) that successful hospices cite "Enrichment Activities" such as the establishment of more in-depth bereavement services as important or key developmental events. They point out that while all hospices provide some degree of bereavement support, new hospices often feel unable to undertake major bereavement service programs. Well-established hospices become more secure and able to enhance or expand services.

Diversity

The diversity and unique nature of a hospice's bereavement service parallels both the unique nature of grief and the individual personalities of hospice programs. And, the nature of the community defines the nature of the hospice program and its services. One of the major factors regarding bereavement services that emerged in this survey was the influence of size upon the delivery of services. Clearly, rural, volunteer-intensive hospices will offer services that are consistent with the community that they serve, and with their limited resources. The wide range in the number of deaths per year (10-900) speaks to the diversity of need in hospice bereavement programs.

Staffing

Setting clear and measurable goals is necessary for the determination of effectiveness or success of services (Osterweis et al., 1984; Lattanzi, 1988). The impression from the varying responses to the survey is that the individual coordinating bereavement services, or the interests of the staff/leadership of the hospice largely shape the delivery of services. With the emergence of Social Work as the primary discipline (36%) involved in the coordination of bereavement services, the need for models that are clinically based and supervised but not pathologizing arises.

In regards to Bereavement Personnel, it was heartening to see an average of 85% of Bereavement Coordinators salaried at some level and spending an average of 11.5 hours per week on coordination activities. The ratio of over 4 to 1 of volunteers to staff in bereavement care spoke to the practical necessity and benefits of utilizing volunteers in bereavement follow-up. Parkes (1981) has noted the effectiveness of volunteers in providing services to the bereaved. The responsibilities of training, supervision and support are inherent in involvement of volunteers. The challenge is for already overburdened hospice bereavement staff not to develop mentalities of having to directly provide all services themselves. Human beings who are overworked and under stressful demands often take on more responsibility for activities that could easily and appropriately be delegated to other staff, or in this case, volunteers. The most significant roles of staff members in hospice bereavement care center around the assessment process and the supervision and training of volunteers.

Strengths of Services

The great strength of hospice bereavement programs lie in their creativity and in their individual innovation, especially in the face of limited resources (Average = 7% of hospice budget). While there exists a core set of hospice bereavement services, individual hospices offer these services to the degree and in the manner that suits their values and their population. The varying responses to the "Services Provided" item points out the emphasis on different services, e.g., phone calls, visits, correspondence materials, groups, etc. Phone calls by bereavement personnel (88%), and phone calls by the nurse involved prior to the death (83%) were the most prevalent hospice bereavement services. The emphasis on telephone contact has implications for selection and training of personnel and for the evaluation of services. For rural hospices, or for very large programs, telephone contact may be the only realistic alternative. It would seem important to establish criteria, screening methods, time frames and protocols that would allow for maximizing the potential of a telephone bereavement contact.

The survey clearly showed that hospice bereavement programs make few referrals to outside counseling or psychotherapy (6%). It seems important that with limited resources hospices allocate them to the persons most receptive to the model of supportive intervention. There is a serious question about the appropriateness of hospice involvement in intensive grief therapy, or in clinical interventions with persons who fall outside of the broad range of what is considered "normal grief."

Priorities

Any bereavement service priority that a hospice develops, whether visits, phone calls, or correspondence, should optimally be focused on consistency, excellence, ongoing evaluation and consumer feedback about that service.

While the surveys showed that the service estimated to be provided to the largest number of bereaved persons was phone calls by either bereavement personnel (89%) or the nurse involved prior to the death (83%), an estimated 83% also receive visits by bereavement personnel. When programs were asked to name their top service priorities, "visits to the bereaved" was most frequently listed as the first priority (47%). An additional 24% listed phone calls to the bereaved as the first priority. The second program priority of the collective sample of 232 responses was phone calls to the bereaved (24%). "Group Meetings" was ranked as the third bereavement priority (21.5%), and was also the service that most bereavement programs indicated they would wish to increase "if time and money were no object" (31%). This data indicates a need for hospices to formally determine their service priorities and to devote time and other resources in a way that is consistent with those priorities. Success and evaluation become more possible when goals are defined and priorities are named.

Another issue related to priorities is the identification of which bereaved persons will receive services. Although 26.5% of the hospices responded that "all" bereaved individuals received services, and another 33% reported "personal contact with all" bereaved persons, some programs with large populations may find this goal difficult. The norm seems to be to extend services to all bereaved persons, with the individual's need and desire for the services becoming the determining factors. The "High Risk" only approach does not seem prevalent among hospices. The value of assessing risk then relates to determining the type and degree of services that are best for the bereaved individual, and to identifying which referrals and other resources would be most helpful.

In addition, effective and comprehensive training programs are a priority (Lindstrom, 1983). Hospices need to examine the scope and relevance of their training programs as they relate to the real needs of care providers and volunteers. The survey findings that most hospices offer initial general training for all caregivers (N = 237, 93%) averaging 16 hours indicates the general fulfillment of that Hospice Standard of Care. While only 10% of the respondents offered specific additional bereavement training, 5% did offer ongoing training for bereavement personnel. Training sets the tone and framework for the delivery of services and can be one of the hospice's most supportive and essential efforts (Lattanzi, 1983).

Further Questions — Risk Factors

The survey created as many questions as it examined. Are adequate and consistent clinical criteria being used to evaluate the responses and coping patterns of individuals? Are hospices thoughtfully considering possible measures for risk potential?

A recommendation based upon the findings of this survey would be for the study and standardization of tools that measure risk. Gabriel and Kirschling (1988) have developed a helpful framework for hospices to evaluate assessment tools. More studies need to examine the optimal ways to identify bereaved persons who are most at risk, or who need additional intervention.

There may be a role for a national task force or committee to examine various risk assessment tools and to make recommendations of those most useful in hospice settings. Standardization of bereavement risk assessment could create a significant body of data to examine, and could hopefully lead to a higher quality of clinical care and service. This suggestion is not made to minimize cultural or programmatic differences or to diminish the autonomy and creativity that are the hallmarks of hospice programming. Rather, this approach may offer hospice programs several effective alternatives to evaluate in the context of their own needs. It also could represent a model of interdisciplinary cooperation that would limit "reinventing the wheel," and encourage the collection of valuable data.

Obstacles and Opportunities

The most prevalent obstacle reported in the survey was the lack of staff time. This could be related to the fact that many of the persons coordinating bereavement services have multiple roles and responsibilities in the hospice program. Directly related, the second major barrier reported was the lack of personnel. Hospices find it difficult to fund bereavement positions, or to allocate sufficient time to their coordination. Unless bereavement services are given specific program priority, they will continue to suffer from a scarcity of resources. Just as hospice services have an orientation rooted in mental health prevention, hospices also need to recognize that bereavement services are largely preventive and supportive by definition. At the present time, this reality means few financial resources will be available through reimbursement.

Areas for Growth

A striking reality that the survey pointed out was the fact that very few hospices (N = 28, 10.5% of total survey sample) utilize the services of students. While some hospices may not have appropriately trained persons to supervise various disciplines of students, it appears that many have probably not developed the necessary relationships with local universities or colleges.

Students are invaluable resources and cost-effective providers of services. Beyond that, they carry with them into their professional work the valuable lessons and experience of hospice care. Hospices could find great resources of energy, talent, expertise, creativity and enthusiasm in the utilization of student interns and student practicum persons from a wide variety of disciplines. An innovative example was the Hospice of Metro Denver's cooperation with dental students in a special pilot project.

One of the glaring deficiencies shown by the survey is the lack of participation in research (None = 94%) or data collection efforts (None = 60%). Although the reimbursement of hospice care legitimizes our efforts, data collection and research activities are necessary to insure quality and clinical excellence. The patients and families with whom we work deserve the best possible care and services that are born out of tested clinical knowledge and experience. Hospice bereavement care is at a developmental stage where soft assumptions or myths are no longer acceptable. Data collection and research are the keys to the continued exploration of the effectiveness of all hospice services.

The seeds of hospice grew from a medical care system that was inattentive and presumptive concerning the needs of dying persons and their families. The era of paternalism in medical care is passing. Hospices must remember the tradition of advocacy that was a central value in the emergence and continuation of their services. Advocacy as it relates to dying persons and their families and to quality of care issues demands diligence in continuing to examine all approaches to care. Refinement and improvement then becomes the necessary norm of hospice care.

REFERENCES

de St. Aubin, M. & Lund, D.A. (1986). A critical test of specific hospice objectives for family caregivers. *The Hospice Journal, 2*(2), 1-18.

Lattanzi, M. E. (1982). Hospice bereavement services: Creating networks of support. *Family and Community Health, 5*(3), 54-63.

Lattanzi, M.E. (1988). Does bereavement follow-up achieve anything: The voice of clinical and personal experience. *The Journal of Palliative Care, 4*(1 & 2), 81-83.

Lattanzi, M.E. (1983). Learning and caring: Education and training concerns. In C.A. Corr & D.M. Corr (Eds.), *Hospice care: Principles and practice* (pp. 223-236). New York: Springer Publishing Co.

Lindstrom, B. (1983). Operating a hospice bereavement program. In C.A. Corr & D.M. Corr (Eds.), *Hospice care: Principles and practice* (pp. 266-277). New York: Springer Publishing Co.

National Hospice Organization (1980). *Standards of hospice program of care.* McLean, VA: National Hospice Organization.

Osterweis, M. (1984). Bereavement intervention programs. In M. Osterweis, F. Solomon & M. Green (Eds.), *Bereavement: Reactions, consequences, and care* (pp. 239-279). Washington, D.C.: National Academy Press.

O'Toole, D. (1985). *Bridging the bereavement gap.* Lapeer, MI: Lapeer Area Hospice.

Parkes, C.M. (1981). Evaluation of a bereavement service. *Journal of Preventive Psychiatry, 1,* 179-188.

Simson, S. & Wilson, L.B. (1986). Strategies for success: An examination of the organizational development of early hospice programs. *The Hospice Journal, 2*(2) 19-39.

Assessing Grief
Among the Bereaved Elderly:
A Review of Existing Measures

Roy M. Gabriel
Jane Marie Kirschling

SUMMARY. The assessment of grief in the elderly, bereaved population has received much attention in the research and clinical literature. Existing instruments vary widely in their complexity, the extent of their theoretical base and in the evidence of their reliability and validity for their intended uses. In this article, the authors describe important principles for the assessment of grief, and present a rating instrument for use in comparing potential measures for this assessment. Nine of the most widely cited measures are reviewed using this process. Their variations along critical dimensions of assessment quality are clearly demonstrated. The general status of available measures, and recommendations for using this rating process in specific clinical settings are discussed.

INTRODUCTION

Hospice care continues for the family into the bereavement period (National Hospice Organization, 1980). While the specific type of services that are offered vary, there is an underlying need for assessment of the bereaved family members' ability to cope, their stress levels, and available support (Lattanzi, 1982). The need for assessing client progress has also been stressed by Demi (1984).

The focus of this article is on the assessment of grief in adult

Roy M. Gabriel, PhD, is affiliated with Northwest Regional Educational Laboratory, Portland, OR. Jane Marie Kirschling, RN, DNS, is Associate Professor, Department of Family Nursing, The Oregon Health Sciences University, Portland, OR.

family members, with two underlying purposes. First, we evaluate the existing measures of adult grief for their potential usefulness in clinical settings in assessing older persons' grief. Secondly, we introduce a rating instrument for clinicians to use for their own evaluations of possible measures of adult grief. The emphasis on older persons is due to both the demographics of our population and the likelihood of experiencing death with age. This emphasis is not intended to minimize the experiences of younger persons, but to explore the work that has been done with the elderly since measurement issues arise as part of normal aging.

The existing measures of adult grief were identified through an extensive review of the literature on widowhood. Approximately 100 research-based articles dating back to the early 1970s were reviewed in order to systematically identify what measures were being used with bereaved adults. In addition, books on hospice care were reviewed to determine what issues and methods, if any, were addressed in relation to grief assessment.

This literature review yielded more than 20 measures that researchers commonly used. These measures generally fell into one of two categories: (1) measures of grief and (2) measures of depression. After this initial process of identification of measures the authors decided to evaluate only the measures of grief in this study. This decision was based on the fact that while the behavior exhibited and distress experienced by grieving individuals is somewhat similar to that of clinically depressed persons there are meaningful differences between the behaviors and experiences of the bereaved and clinically depressed persons. For example, "Most grieving people do not report gross motor retardation or suicidal thoughts" (Osterweis, Solomon, & Green, 1984, p. 19).

A variety of measures of depression have been used with bereaved populations. Some of these include: The Hopkins Symptom Checklist (Degorgatis, Lipman, Rickels, Uhlenhuth, & Covi, 1974) which was used by Murphy (1984); Zung Self-Rating Depression Scale (Zung & Zung, 1986) which was used by Valanis and Yeaworth (1982) and Dimond, Lund, and Castera (1987); and, the Goldberg General Health Questionnaire (Goldberg, 1979) which was used by Vachon, Rogers, Lyall, Lancee, Sheldon, and Freeman (1982). Clinicians interested in learning more about the depression measures and some of the issues related to measuring depression in older persons will find thorough treatment in the work of Kane and Kane (1981) and Brink (1986).

This sharpened focus left us with nine existing measures of grief. Alphabetically, they are: (1) *Adjustment Scale* (Carey, 1977; Carey, 1979-1980); (2) *Bereavement Items* (Jacobs, 1987; Jacobs, Kasl, Ostfeld, Berkman, & Charpentier, 1986; Jacobs, Kasl, Ostfeld, Berkman, Kosten, & Charpentier, 1987; Jacobs, Kosten, Kasl, Ostfeld, Berkman, & Charpentier, 1987-1988); (3) *Boulder County Hospice Bereavement Assessment Referral* (Lattanzi & Coffelt, 1979); (4) *Grief Experience Inventory* (Sanders, 1980-1981 & 1982-1983; Sanders, Mauger, & Strong, 1979); (5) *Grief Resolution Index* (Remondet & Hannson, 1987); (6) *Impact of Event Scale* (Horowitz, Wilner, & Alvarez, 1979; Zilberg, Weiss, & Horowitz, 1982); (7) *Present Feelings about Loss* (Singh & Raphael, 1981); (8) *Texas Inventory of Grief* (Faschingbauer, DeVaul, & Zisook, 1977); and (9) *Texas Revised Inventory of Grief* (Faschingbauer, 1981; Faschingbauer, Zisook, & DeVaul, 1987).

The Boulder County Hospice has emerged in the past 10 years as a model for a number of hospice programs across the country. Although there is no way to know the extent of the use of the Boulder County Hospice Bereavement Assessment Referral, the authors elected to include it in this review in order to present the reader with an assessment tool that has been used in clinical practice.

There were two additional measures that emerged from the literature review. Specific information on these measures was not available at the time of this review, however, so they could not be included. The measures were the Bereavement Experience Questionnaire (Demi, 1984) and a list of factors to consider in high-risk assessment (Lindstrom, 1983). The authors acknowledge that additional measures may be available that were not located through the review process.

The remainder of this article is organized into three sections. They include: a description of the rating instrument and procedures used to evaluate the nine measures of adult grief, the actual evaluation and description of the nine measures, and discussion of the findings from the evaluation along with implications for future use of the rating instrument by practicing clinicians.

THE RATING INSTRUMENT

In attempting to assess the extent of grief in elderly, bereaved individuals, several important aspects of available measurement tools must be considered. In this section, we identify seven major areas of consideration, each operationalized by specific questions. The list of issues presented here is not unique. Many are discussed at length in the published standards for educational and psychological tests developed cooperatively by the American Psychological Association, the American Educational Research Association, and the National Council on Measurement in Education. Grief assessment in hospice care shares many of these concerns and presents specific challenges along many of these critical dimensions.

We propose seven criteria for screening and judging available or recommended assessment procedures. As noted in our introductory comments, we employ these criteria in evaluating measures of grief found in the current literature, and discuss the results in the next section. We also suggest that clinicians in need of such measurement tools in their own work adopt this rating framework to ensure that the measure they select meets their needs and fits their context of use.

The seven dimensions are discussed below, along with a sampling of good practices related to each. A sample of the rating instrument itself, complete with specific questions relating each of the seven evaluative dimensions, is given in the Appendix.

1. Validity

While technically existing in many forms, the essential indicator of validity is that the instrument or procedure is measuring what it intends or claims to measure. For example, the assessment of grief in the bereaved family of a hospice patient must truly get at that characteristic, rather than something perhaps related but different such as a more general index of mental health or positive/negative outlook on life. Clear evidence of validity depends upon a clear statement of what is being measured.

Evidence of validity can come from a variety of approaches. In the bereavement literature we examined, there were essentially two types: *construct validity* and *criterion-related validity*. Construct validity is the specification of group differences on the measure of grief, where those groups consist of people who vary in ways hypothetically related to degree of grief (e.g., closeness of relationship with the deceased and years since the loss). Demonstrating that those groups also differ on the measure of grief lends credibility to the validity of that measure. Criterion-related validity is similar, but rather than rely on group discriminations, it establishes a network of interrelationship of scores on the measure of grief with scores on previously-validated measures of other related behaviors or attitudes (e.g., depression).

Both of these approaches are valuable. Generally, ratings will be higher when several independent studies or demonstrations of validity are presented.

2. Reliability

Classically, the reliability of an assessment relates to its consistency. In the literature we examined, there were two general approaches to establishing this aspect of measures of grief: *internal consistency* coefficients and *test-retest* reliabilities. There are many variations of internal consistency measures — split-half, Kuder-Richardson, Cronbach's alpha — but they have one essential feature in common: they arise from a single administration of the instrument to the same sample of individuals. Test-retest measures, on the other hand, involve two assessments on the same sample, separated by a meaningful amount of time.

In general, ratings of the instruments we examined were higher when researchers studied the consistency of their measurement tools using both of these approaches. However, the preference for one approach over the other depends upon the intended use of the instrument (see discussion on "Breadth of Application" which follows). If it is to be used for a single point in time assessment, internal consistency coefficients are probably sufficient. If, however, it will be used to measure change in an individual's grief over time, the test-retest approach is preferred.

An issue related to reliability is the consistency in interpretation of its results. The key point here is that the technique must have sufficient clarity and objectivity to not produce meaningfully different interpretations when used on the same person under similar conditions.

3. Administration

The conditions and procedures under which the assessment tool is used must be specified. The more complex instruments require specific training to use and interpret properly. Others are self-explanatory and can be readily employed by volunteers as well as trained clinicians. Some may be rather time-consuming to use, possibly involving conferring with several people in order to complete. Others may be very brief, but less thorough. At a minimum, the instructions or manual accompanying the assessment tool ought to be explicit about administration conditions. And again, these requirements must fit the intended use.

4. Breadth of Application

The population, conditions and intended uses of the assessment tool must bear a reasonable match to those in which it was developed. Population and conditions refer to any factors which can be expected to affect the assessment. Age group, cultural background, socioeconomic level, etc., of the population on which the procedures were developed may be an important qualifier to its potential application. Similarly, the intended use is a critical specification. It is one thing to use an assessment procedure to determine which families or family members are in need of supporting services. It is quite another to try to diagnose specifically what services they need or whether they have improved significantly as a result of those services. At a minimum, these important limiting conditions must be specified to future users. More desirably, they should be replicated with other populations, conditions or users to demonstrate a broader field of application.

In general, instruments we reviewed were rated more highly when authors were clear about how the instrument could be used, and they had been used with a variety of populations and under conditions which represent important variations to hospice applications.

5. Theoretical Basis

The conceptual and theoretical framework under which the instrument or procedure was developed is an important feature of the assessment tool. Most basically, it provides another evaluative screen to use in considering its use. That is, if a hospice caregiver does not agree with the philosophy underlying the instrument, he/she probably will not find its results very useful. Secondarily, a clear theoretical link to a philosophy of hospice care will provide important assistance in judging other aspects of the technique's usefulness, for example, its validity and the breadth of applicability. Least desirable are those instruments or diagnostic tools which have no apparent theoretical base.

6. Information Yield

What does the result of using the procedure tell you? A minimal information yield might be a single, global indicator of the extent of grief in the individual being measured. If such an indicator meets other criteria discussed — is sufficiently valid, matches the intended use, etc. — this may be just what is needed. If more specific information is required — such as greater detail in particular aspects of grieving, likely consequent behaviors or implications for the type of support services needed — instruments with a richer array of subscales and scoring procedures may be desired. Finally, the availability of normative data from the instrument's development and use enables future users to compare their client population with a larger, representative group of bereaved persons.

7. Accessibility

This refers to one of the more practical issues in our rating instrument: is the instrument or procedure, along with the necessary background information, easy to obtain? In our search of the literature, we experienced wide variations in this. Some of the instruments were included as appendices in the research articles which

presented evidence of reliability, validity, etc. Others required telephone calls to the original authors. Some of these resulted in a dis-
couraging series of dead ends — hence the inclusion of only nine
instruments in this review.

Other considerations related to this are cost and copyright considerations. Are there copyright issues? Is there any cost for its use,
explicit or hidden? We found that often this information was not
readily available.

RESULTS OF THE RATING PROCESS

The results of our ratings of the nine instruments selected for this
review are summarized in Tables 1 and 2 in this section. In Table 1,
we synthesize a common set of information found on each instrument in three general categories. First, a description of the instrument, its length, any subscales it contains and the sample(s) on
which it was validated are provided. Secondly, the specific types of
reliability and validity evidence presented in the references we examined are noted. Finally, amidst all the supporting references to
many of these instruments, we indicate the specific article or source
from which the instrument can be obtained.

In Table 2, the results of our ratings of the nine instruments are
presented. The ratings on a 0- to 4-point scale are provided for all
but four of the questions on the instrument shown in the Appendix.
These four questions were omitted for this review because they are
entirely dependent upon the particular clinical context in which they
would be used. The current authors could not effectively rate any of
these instruments on whether "the model underlying the instrument
is consistent with yours" (question 12), for example.

Scores on each of the seven major dimensions ("Validity," "Reliability," etc.) are also tallied in Table 2, following the items com-
prising each dimension. No "grand total" score for each instrument
as a whole is presented in the table. The current authors feel strongly
that simply adding up the totals for each dimension does not comprise a meaningful evaluative composite of each instrument. There
will be no single, universally superior instrument arising from a
review conducted at this general a level. Instead, potential users are

encouraged to focus in on the dimensions most important to them in using this rating procedure to select an instrument. For example, if strong evidence of validity is the most important characteristic, the Texas Revised Inventory of Grief (TRIG) is among the most highly rated of the nine and would be a good choice on this basis. If, however, ease of administration is a primary criterion, the TRIG is one of the least desirable.

DISCUSSION

As the information provided in Table 1 and the evaluative results presented in Table 2 are examined, the authors conclude this review with some observations about the status of grief assessment instruments in the field and some recommendations for use of the rating instrument for specific assessment purposes.

The instruments we reviewed can be described along a series of dichotomies. First, they were either very short and simple or quite long and factorially complex. Carey's (1977) Adjustment Scale (AS), for example, consisted of only eight simple, easily interpretable questions. Reliability and validity data were minimal, but the AS represents well that set of instruments which can be easily used by clinicians or volunteers. At the other extreme perhaps is the Grief Experience Inventory (GEI) with 135 items, factor analyzed to 18 overlapping subscales and correlated with the subscales of the MMPI. It may be the most extensive research tool, but requires serious study before being used in many clinical settings.

Few of the instruments present sufficient reliability and validity data to warrant use in measuring change or progress of individuals in dealing with their grief. The Bereavement Items (BI) combined with the Depression scale of the Center for Epidemiological Studies (CES-D) offers some potential here, particularly if the promising research of Jacobs et al. (1987) continues.

The Boulder Grief Assessment materials provide little primary data evidencing reliability and validity of their bereavement assessment referral form, but their supporting materials indicate the importance of potential users establishing these standards for their own use. In some contrast is the Present Feelings About Loss

TABLE 1. Information on Existing Measures of Grief

Title/Description of Measure	Validity	Reliability	How to Obtain Materials
Adjustment Scale (AS) 8 items, Sample included 41 widowers and 78 widows (mean age 56 years) and 68 married people (mean age 56 years). Solie & Fielder (1987-1988) have used the AS.	Correlated highly with Borstein-Clayton measure of depression. Construct validity comparing widowed and married subjects, forewarned verses not forewarned.	Split-half reliability = .86.	Items listed in Carey (1977).

Bereavement Items (BI) 38 items/18 on grief and 20 items, Center for Epidemiological Studies-Depression Scale (CES-D) (Radloff, 1977). Sample included 150 bereaved and 68 non-bereaved adults (age range 46-80). Yields 3 scales: Numbness-Disbelief, Separation Anxiety, and CES-D. Intended use: Study of relationship of bereavement to ill health.	Construct validity contrasting early bereaved, late bereaved, and non-bereaved on all 3 scales. Comparisons among groups and over time. CES-D correlates significantly with a number of the depression and mood scales and also discriminates between groups (Corcoran & Fisher, 1987)	Internal consistency: Numbness-Disbelief .73 to .90 and Separation Anxiety .84 to .86. CES-D split-half range from .77 to .92. Test-retest range from .32 to .67 depending on time interval (Corcoran & Fisher, 1987)	Items provided in Jacobs et al. (1987-1988) and Jacobs (1987).

TABLE 1 (continued)

Title/Description of Measure	Validity	Reliability	How to Obtain Materials
Boulder County Hospice Bereavement Assessment Referral (BAR) Demographic, death related information and 13 items.	Not available. Refers to preliminary work of Dr. Colin Murray Parkes (1976) in conjunction with the Royal Victoria Hospital Palliative Care Unit, Montreal. Lattanzi and Coffert (1979) state "that replication and cross validation of information are important responsibilities in examining the effects and effectiveness of Hospice bereavement followup services" (p. 27).		Measure in Lattanzi & Coffelt (1979) Write Boulder County Hospice, 2825 Marine St., Boulder, CO 80303. Cost $

Grief Experience Inventory (GEI) 135 items. Sample included 135 adults (e.g. college students and a community of bereaved persons). Early bereavement group (N = 102) had a mean age of 52, they were identified through obituaries. Yields 18 overlapping subscales. Intended use is research. Ferrell (1985) and Kirschling (1988) have used the BEI.	Extensive correlations with other scales, such as MMPI, are reported in the manual (range -1.0 to +1.0). Construct validity comparing groups (e.g., nature of loss).	Internal consistency of 18 scales ranged from .23 to .84. Test-retest of 9 weeks and 18 months ranged from .18 to .87.	Measure provided in Sanders et al. (1979). Write Consulting Psychologist Press, 577 College Ave., CA 94306. Cost $10 Manual and $11 basic materials.

TABLE 1 (continued)

Title/Description of Measure	Validity	Reliability	How to Obtain Materials
Grief Resolution Index (GRI) 7 items. Sample included 75 widows, 60-90 years old, mean length of widowhood 10.3 years. Intended use is identification of individuals who continue to experience bereavement related distress.	Scores on GRI broadly related to 14 other measures of coping and adjustment.	Cronbach's alpha = .87; Factor loading .67 to .84.	Items provided in Remondet & Hansson (1987).

Impact of Event Scale (IES) 15 items. Three samples included 66 adults who sought psychotherapy as a result of reaction to serious life event (34 bereaved) (age range 20-75) and 72 bereaved adult children (mean age 31) in two samples. Yields three scales: Total Stress Scale, Intrusion and Avoidance. Intended uses research and individual assessment.

Discriminant validity. Groups experiencing different levels of severity of stress events were found to be significantly different. Pre-post comparisons of groups before and after therapy.

Split-half reliability .86; Cronbach's alpha: Intrusion .78 and Avoidance .82. Correlation between two scales .42. One week test-retest with 25 adult students: Total Stress Score .87, Intrusion .89 and Avoidance .79.

Measure provided in Corcoran & Fisher (1987)

43

TABLE 1 (continued)

Title/Description of Measure	Validity	Reliability	How to Obtain Materials
Present Feelings about Loss (PFL) 16 items. Sample included 44 subjects who had a next-of-kin die in a rail disaster in Australia (age ranged 37-59). Yields 3 scales: Affective Distress, Inability to Give Up Lost Object and Inability to Return to Normal Function. Intended use is as an interview protocol for individual assessment.	Construct validity comparing groups (e.g., intervention vs. non-intervention, adequate vs. inadequate support, and relationship with deceased).	Not available.	The interview protocol is provided in Singh & Raphael (1981). It is not a paper and pencil test.

44

Texas Inventory Grief (TIG)
7 items. Sample included 57
patients in a psychiatric
outpatient clinic who had
lost one or more first-
degree relatives. Intended
use is as an eventual
screening tool with
additional research. The
measure has evolved into the
Texas Revised Inventory of
Grief (described below).

Construct
validity:
Groups
experiencing
recent deaths
scored
significantly
higher on
total score.

Internal
consistency
(split-half)
analysis,
using
iterative
scale
development
technique.
Average inter-
item
correlation.
67. Split-
half
reliability
.81.

Items
provided
in
Fasch-
ingbauer
et al.
(1977).

TABLE 1 (continued)

Title/Description of Measure	Validity	Reliability	How to Obtain Materials
Texas Revised Inventory of Grief (TRIG) 33 items. Sample of 260 bereaved persons (mean age 38). Replication sample of 328 persons (mean age 33). Yields 2 scales: Past Behavior and Present Feelings. Intended use is individual assessment (sensitive to measuring change). Gallagher et al. (1983) and Farberow et al. (1987) have used the TRIG with a sample of 199 bereaved spouse (mean age 70).	Construct validity of scales assessed using variety of group discriminations (e.g., age of deceased, sex of survivor, and spouses vs. other relationship).	Both split-half and coefficient alpha's are provided. Past Behavior range from .74 to .87 and Present Feeling range from .82 to .89.	Measure provided in Faschingbauer et al. (1987) or Write Dr. Faschingbauer, 5015 Montrose, Houston, TX 77006. Cost $30 includes manual, scoring templet and 50 forms.

(PFAL) instrument. It is simply a set of 16 questions used in an interview protocol, with little supporting evidence of reliability and validity and little direction to potential users.

The current authors have found the instrument presented in the Appendix a concise, useful tool for discriminating among available instruments for assessing grief in the bereaved. We recommend that it be used by a team of staff, each of whom brings a different perspective to the task of assessing grief in a specified population or context. The authors here represent two varying perspectives — one whose training is in measures in a variety of applied contexts, the other a nursing clinician and researcher. Our ratings varied somewhat as we proceeded through the dimensions of the instrument, but they were reconciled fairly quickly through comparative analyses of various measures in this review.

A second suggestion for use of the instrument is that it not be used on a single measurement tool. It is necessarily a comparative device. We felt more comfortable in our ratings when we were able to compare those that we had given several other instruments with the one we were currently rating.

Finally, and in summary, our purpose was to provide a brief, but systematic, review of available instruments for the assessment of grief in the bereaved, elderly population. In the process, we developed what we hope is a useful set of principles and rating instrument for clinicians to consider in their own setting.

TABLE 2. Application of Rating Instrument with Existing Measures of Grief

	VALIDITY				RELIABILITY			ADMINISTRATION		
	#1 Clear Definition?	#2 Related Behaviors?	#3 Evidence of Validity?	Total	#4 Consistent Results?	#5 Easily Interpretable?	Total	#6 Minimal/No Training?	#7 Time Required?	Total
Adjustment Scale (1977)	2	1	1	4	2	3	5	4	4	8
Bereavement Items/ CES–D (1986)	4	3	3	10	4	4	8	4	3	7
Boulder Grief Assessment (1979)	1	0	0	1	0	4	4	4	4	8
Grief Experience Inventory (1979)	3	3	2	8	3	1[b]	4	3	1	4
Grief Resolution Index (1987)	2	3	2	7	2	4	6	4	4	8
Impact of Event Scale (1979)	4	0	4	8	4	4	8	4	4	8
Present Feelings About Loss (1981)	3	1	2	6	0	3	3	4	4	8
Texas Inventory Grief (1977)	3	0	1	4	3	4	7	4	4	8
Texas Revised Grief Inventory (1981)	4	2	4	10	4	4	8	4	2	6

[a] Little work has been done with bereaved elderly persons.
[b] Complexity of interpretation increased with number of items.

BREADTH			THEORY		INFORMATION YIELD			ACCESSIBILITY	
#8 Variety of Populations?	#9 Appropriate Use?	Total	#11 Theoretical Model?	Total	#13 Normative Data?	#14 Subscales?	Total	#16 Materials Available?	Total
0	4	4	0	0	0	1	1	3	3
3	3	6	4	4	3	3	6	3	3
0	4	4	0	0	0	1	1	2	2
3[a]	3	6	3	3	3	3	6	2[c]	2
0	4	4	2	2	0	1	1	3	3
3[a]	3[d]	6	3	3	3[a]	3	6	4	4
1	2	3	2	2	0	2	2	2	2
1	1	2	3	3	0	1	1	3	3
3[a]	4	7	3	3	4	4	8	4	4

[c] Items/measures not published in literature, only available in manual.
[d] Not developed specifically for bereaved persons.

REFERENCES

Brink, T.L. (1986). *Clinical gerontology: A guide to assessment and intervention*. NY: Haworth Press.

Carey, R.G. (1977). The widowed: A year later. *Journal of Counseling Psychology*, *24*, 125-131.

Carey, R.G. (1979-1980). Weathering widowhood: Problems and adjustment of the widowed during the first year. *Omega*, *10*, 163-174.

Corcoran, K., & Fisher, J. (1987). *Measures for clinical practice: A sourcebook*. NY: The Free Press.

Demi, A.S. (1984). Hospice bereavement program: Trends and issues. In S.H. Schraff (Ed.), *Hospice: The nursing perspective* (pp. 131-151). NY: National League for Nursing (Pub. No. 20-1967).

Derogatis, L.R., Lipman, R.S., Rickels, K., Uhlenhuth, E.H., & Covi, L. (1974). The Hopkins Symptom Checklist (HSCL): A measure of primary symptom dimensions. *Pharmacopsychiatry*, *7*, 79-110.

Dimond, M., Lund, D.A., & Caserta, M.S. (1987). The role of social support in the first two years of bereavement in an elderly sample. *The Gerontologist*, *27*, 599-604.

Farberow, N.L., Gallagher, D.E., Gilweski, M.J., & Thompson, L.W. (1987). An examination of the early impact of bereavement on psychological distress in survivors of suicide. *The Gerontologist*, *27*, 592-598.

Faschingbauer, T.R. (1981). *Texas Revised Inventory of Grief Manual*. Houston, TX: Honeycomb Publishing (5015 Montrose Blvd, Houston, TX 77006).

Faschingbauer, T.R., DeVaul, R.A., & Zisook, S. (1977). Development of the Texas Inventory of Grief. *American Journal of Psychiatry*, *134*, 696-698.

Faschingbauer, T.R., Zisook, S., & DeVaul, R. (1987). The Texas Revised Inventory of Grief. In S. Zisook (Ed.), *Biopsychosocial aspects of bereavement* (pp. 111-124). Washington, D.C.: American Psychiatric Press, Inc.

Ferrell, B.R. (1985). Cancer deaths and bereavement outcomes: Home versus hospital. *The American Journal of Hospice Care*, *2*(4), 18-23.

Gallagher, D.E., Breckenridge, J.N., Thompson, L.W., & Peterson, J.A. (1983). Effects of bereavement on indicators of mental health in elderly widows and widowers. *Journal of Gerontology*, *38*, 565-571.

Goldberg, D. (1972). *The detection of psychiatric illness by questionnaire, a technique for the identification of nonpsychotic psychiatric illness: Institute of Psychiatry Maudsley Monographs 21*. London: Oxford University Press.

Horowitz, M., Wilner, N., & Alvarez, W. (1979). Impact of Event Scale: A measure of subjective stress. *Psychosomatic Medicine*, *41*, 209-218.

Jacobs, S.C. (1987). Measures of the psychological distress of bereavement. In S. Zisook (Ed.), *Biopsychosocial distress of bereavement* (pp. 127-155). Washington, D.C.: American Psychiatric Press.

Jacobs, S., Kasl, S., Ostfeld, A., Berkman, L., & Charpentier, P. (1986). The measurement of grief: Age and sex variation. *British Journal of Medical Psychology, 59,* 305-310.

Jacobs, S.C., Kasl, S.V., Ostfeld, A.M., Berkman, L., Kosten, T.R., & Charpentier, P. (1987). The measurement of grief: Bereaved versus non-bereaved. *The Hospice Journal, 2*(4), 21-36.

Jacobs, S.C., Kosten, T.R., Kasl, S.V., Ostfeld, A.M., Berkman, L., & Charpentier, P. (1987-1988). Attachment theory and multiple dimensions of grief. *Omega, 18,* 41-52.

Kane, R.A., & Kane, R.L. (1981). *Assessing the elderly: A practical guide to measurement.* Lexington, MA: Lexington Books.

Kirschling, J.M. (1988). Analysis of Bugen's Model of Grief. *The Hospice Journal,* 55-75.

Lattanzi, M.E. (1982). Hospice bereavement services: Creating networks of support. *Family and Community Health,* November, 54-63.

Lattanzi, M., & Coffelt, D. (1979). *Bereavement care manual.* Boulder, CO: Boulder County Hospice, Inc.

Lindstrom, B. (1983). Operating a hospice bereavement program. In C.A. Corr & D.M. Corr (Eds.), *Hospice care principles and practice* (pp. 266-277). NY: Springer.

Murphy, S.A. (1984). Stress levels and health status of victims of natural disaster. *Research in Nursing and Health, 7,* 205-215.

National Hospice Organization (1980). *Standings for a hospice program of care.* Washington, D.C.: National Hospice Organization.

Osterweis, M., Solomon, F., & Green, M. (1984). *Bereavement reactions consequences, and care.* Washington, D.C.: National Academy Press.

Parkes, C.M. (1976). *Royal Victoria Hospital manual on palliative care.* Montreal, Canada: Royal Victoria Hospital Palliative Care Unit.

Radloff, L.S. (1977). The CES-D Scale: A self-report depression scale for research in the general population. *Applied Psychological Measurement, 1,* 385-401.

Remondet, J.H., & Hansson, R.O. (1987). Assessing a widow's grief—a short index. *Journal of Gerontological Nursing, 13*(4), 31-34.

Sanders, C.M. (1980-1981). Comparison of younger and older spouses in bereavement outcome. *Omega, 11,* 217-232.

Sanders, C.M. (1982-1983). Effects of sudden vs. chronic illness death on bereavement outcomes. *Omega, 13,* 227-241.

Sanders, C.M., Mauger, P.A., & Strong, P.N. (1979). *A manual for the Grief Experience Inventory.*

Singh, B., & Raphael, B. (1981). Postdiseaster morbidity of the bereaved: A possible role for preventive psychiatry? *The Journal of Nervous and Mental Disease, 169,* 203-212.

Solie, L.J., & Fielder, L.J. (1987-1988). The relationship between sex role identity and a widow's adjustment to the loss of a spouse. *Omega, 18,* 33-40.

Vachon, M.L.S., Rogers, J., Lyall, A., Lancee, W.J., Sheldon, A.R., & Freeman, S.J.J. (1982). Predictors and correlates of adaptation to conjugal bereavement. *American Journal of Psychiatry, 139,* 998-1002.

Valanis, B.G., & Yeaworth, R. (1982). Ratings of physical and mental health in the older bereaved. *Research in Nursing and Health, 5,* 137-146.

Zilberg, N.J., Weiss, D.S., & Horowitz, M.J. (1982). Impact of Event Scale: A cross-validation study and some empirical evidence supporting a conceptual model of stress response syndromes. *Journal of Consulting and Clinical Psychology, 50,* 407-414.

Zung, W.W.K., & Zung, E.M. (1986). Use of the Zung Self-Rating Depression Scale in the elderly. In T.L. Brink (Ed.), *Clinical gerontology: A guide to assessment and intervention* (pp. 137-147). NY: Haworth Press.

APPENDIX

Rating Instrument for Measures of Grief in Hospice Care

4 – Very Good
3 – Good
2 – Fair
1 – Poor
0 – Unavailable/Not Addressed

Criteria		*Rating*			
	0	1	2	3	4

VALIDITY

1. Is there a clear definition of what's being measured?
2. Are related behaviors specified?
3. Is there empirical evidence of validity?

RELIABILITY

4. Is there evidence of consistency of results
5. Are results easily interpretable in clinical settings?

Criteria	Rating				
	0	1	2	3	4

ADMINISTRATION

6. Can it be used with little or no training?
7. Can it be administered in a short time period assuming established rapport with the respondents?

BREADTH OF APPLICATION

8. Has it been used with a variety of populations?
9. Is there information about the appropriate uses of the measure (e.g., group vs. individual, clinical diagnosis vs. assessing change over time)?
10. 'Do the conditions fit your context?

THEORETICAL ORIENTATION

11. Is there a theoretical/conceptual model framing the nature of the questions?
12. 'Is the model underlying the instrument consistent with yours?

INFORMATION YIELD

13. Are there normative data to compare your results with?
14. Are there reliable subscales which provide more specific information than simply a total score?
15. 'Is the information provided clear and sufficient for your needs?

	Rating				
Criteria	0	1	2	3	4

ASSESSIBILITY

16. Are the needed materials (e.g., the instrument, scoring procedures, background technical information, etc.) available to clinicians?
17. ¹Are there costs or copyright limitations which may prohibit your intended use?

---

1. These questions will not be rated in this review. They depend entirely upon the clinical setting for which instruments are being considered. They are important questions for clinicians to consider, however, so they are included in the rating instrument.

Analysis of Bugen's
Model of Grief

Jane Marie Kirschling

Hospice care in the United States offers families an array of services that traditionally have not been available. These services include, but are not limited to, the availability of a nurse 24 hours a day to assist the family in caring for the terminally ill person at home, the availability of trained volunteers to provide the family with respite, and the availability of bereavement follow-up. Despite these expanded services the family is confronted with potentially stressful situations. Such situations include assuming the responsibility of caring for the terminally ill member and experiencing the grief associated with the eventual death of the family member.

Although research on the experiences of family members caring for a chronically ill frail elder has rapidly increased in the past decade, a similar emphasis on family members caring for a terminally

Jane Marie Kirschling, RN, DNS, has been clinically active in hospice care and bereavement services for six years. Her research has focused on the widowed and family members caring for a terminally ill elder. She is an associate professor at the Oregon Health Sciences University School of Nursing. Address correspondence to the author at OHSU, 3181 SW Sam Jackson Park Road, EJSN 230, Portland, OR 97201.

Study 2 was funded with a Biomedical Research Support Grant, The Oregon Health Sciences University, Portland, OR. An earlier version of this paper was presented at the National Hospice Organization 1986 Annual Meeting and Symposium, Denver, CO, November 1986.

The author wishes to thank Yvonne Boyer, RN, MS, for her assistance in collecting data; Joan Kessner Austin, RN, DNS, for her contributions to an earlier manuscript; and Bob Flick and Marie Scott Brown, RN, PhD, for their review of this manuscript.

ill elder has not emerged (Kirschling, 1986). This dearth in research exists in spite of the fact that the caregiver is identified as the person who "often has the most to lose by the patient's death" (Abrams, 1974, p. 56).

Death of a family member and the period of time following the death are known to be quite stressful for the survivors. During this period of grief the physical and emotional well-being of the surviving family members may be threatened (Clayton, 1979; Murphy, 1983; Osterweis & Green, 1984; Parkes & Brown, 1972). For some, this period of grief is either prolonged (Vachon, 1979; Parkes & Weiss, 1983) or unresolved (Vachon, Sheldon, Lancee, Lyall, Rogers & Freeman, 1982) which makes these bereaved persons even more vulnerable to physical and/or emotional illness.

It is essential that health care professionals be knowledgeable regarding the caregiving and grief experiences in order that they can intervene effectively with families who are caring, or have cared, for a terminally ill elder. The Committee for the Study of Health Consequences of the Stress of Bereavement (Osterweis & Green, 1984) gave high priority to research aimed at refining and documenting the factors that place a bereaved individual at risk. In addition, it is unclear how the caregiving experience may, or may not, be a risk factor as well. Interestingly, Gerber and colleagues (1975) found that elderly bereaved ($N = 81$) who experienced a lengthy chronic illness of a spouse had poor medical adjustment. With a clear understanding of what constitutes normal grief, the clinician could then identify those variables that have the potential for placing a family member at risk for abnormal grief.

Based on an extensive review of the grief literature, Murphy (1983) concluded that the stage view of bereavement is inadequate to explain the variability found in grief experiences. She further suggested that theories such as the Bugen model (1979) be explored in order to better understand the grief phenomenon. This article reports two studies which explore Bugen's concepts of centrality and preventability. The article is organized into four sections: a description of Bugen's model of grief, a study undertaken with 72 widows and widowers (Study 1), a study undertaken with 40 family caregivers of terminally ill elderly (Study 2), and discussion.

BUGEN'S MODEL OF GRIEF

Bugen's model of grief predicts the intensity and length of the grief process based on two major concepts: the perception of the closeness of the relationship and the extent to which the bereaved perceives that the death could have been prevented. According to Bugen (1979) the term central is applied when the survivor "refers to a person whose presence and importance is so profound that 'I feel I have no life without him'" (p. 35). The survivor may also identify the relationship as a peripheral one. In this case the person's presence is felt but the survivor does not question his or her survival. The term peripheral does not mean that the relationship was of little importance, only that the survivor does not question whether his or her life will go on.

The second major concept of Bugen's model involved the survivor's perception of whether the death was preventable. If the survivor believed the death to be preventable, they may feel that they could have done more to avoid the death. On the other hand, if death is seen as unpreventable survivors should have less guilt since there was nothing more they could do.

Based on these two major concepts, Bugen (1979) predicted four outcomes. If the relationship was central and the survivor believed the death was preventable, then grieving would be intense and prolonged. However, if the relationship was central and the survivor believed the death was not preventable, then grieving would be intense, but brief. When the survivor viewed the relationship as peripheral and the death as preventable, Bugen predicted that grief would be mild and prolonged. In the final outcome when the survivor viewed the relationship as peripheral and the death as not preventable Bugen predicted that grief would be mild and brief.

Although the model appears to make sense clinically, minimal research has been completed on the model. Murphy (1982) and Chenell (1986) measured centrality of the relationship with persons who had experienced a confirmed or presumed death from the Mt. St. Helen's eruption in 1980. Olson (1985) measured the concept of preventability with parents who had experienced a sudden and unexpected infant death. The methods, samples and findings from two research studies using Bugen's model will be described next.

STUDY 1

An exploratory study was undertaken with a sample of the recently widowed in order to test Bugen's model (Kirschling, 1984). Bugen's model predicts four possible grieving conditions based on whether the widow or widower perceives the relationship as central or peripheral and the death as preventable or not. The conditions include whether grief will be brief or prolonged and mild or intense.

The subjects in Study 1 completed the Grief Experience Inventory (GEI) (Sanders, Mauger & Strong, 1979). The GEI is been described as an "objective multidimensional measure of grief which is sensitive to the longitudinal analysis of the process of bereavement" according to the developers (Sanders et al., 1979, p. iv). Due to the unequal number of subjects in each category, the findings on the GEI were explored in relation to the two major concepts, a central/peripheral relationship and preventable/not preventable death. The regression approach to analysis of variance was utilized in order to attempt to statistically control for the unequal cell sizes. Bartlett-Box F tests were also calculated in order to obtain a measure of homogeneity of variance. Research questions were as follows: (1) Are there differences in the grief experience for those who perceived the relationship as central and those who perceived the relationship as peripheral?; and (2) Are there differences in the grief experience for those who perceived the deceased's death as preventable and for those who perceived the death as unpreventable?

Methods and Sample

Potential subjects were identified through county death certificates and they were sent a letter explaining the research. A total of 481 widows and widowers were sent letters describing the study. Of the 481, 72 persons, or 15%, returned a postcard indicating their willingness to participate. After the subjects indicated their willingness to participate they were contacted by telephone to arrange the one-time interview. All of the structured interviews were conducted by the author.

The subjects included 49 widows and 23 widowers from the Midwest. The widows ranged in age from 24 to 83 years with a mean of

62.3. The widowers ranged in age from 24 to 80 with a mean of 65.6. The mean time since death of the spouse for the 72 subjects was 12.6 weeks (range 5 to 20).

Instruments

Forced choice questions were used to measure Bugen's (1979) concepts. Bugen offered a number of expressions that would be associated with a central relationship. The expression that was predicted to be most powerful and indicative of hopelessness was "I feel I have no life without him." A congruent expression, "I wonder how I am going to survive without this person in my life," was used with the 72 widows and widowers (Kirschling, 1984) to operationalize a central relationship. The subjects were asked to select between two expressions. The alternate expression was associated with a peripheral relationship and read "I have a great deal of respect for the deceased and feel an empty void in my life." The subjects were then asked to identify which of the following statements best represented how they felt about the death: "The death could have been prevented" (Preventable), or "The death was not something that could have been prevented" (Not Preventable).

The subjects also completed the Grief Experience Inventory (GEI) (Sanders et al., 1979). Only those scales that had alpha coefficients of .50 or higher with the sample of 72 widows and widowers were included in the data analyses. The alpha coefficients for the 11 scales that were included are as follows: Denial, .60; Atypical Response, .58; Despair, .82; Anger, .66; Guilt, .71; Loss of Control, .53; Rumination, .60; Somatization, .74; Loss of Appetite, .53; Loss of Vigor, .53; and Physical Symptoms, .65.

Findings

The sample is described according to the groups suggested by Bugen's model, followed by the research questions. Figure 1 presents the breakdown of the sample according to the subjects' perceptions of death. For the entire sample, only six subjects identified with the central relationship statement. Only two subjects who identified the relationship as central also perceived the death as preventable. The subjects were women and were 24 and 48 years of

	Central	Peripheral	Total
Preventable	2	10	12
Not Preventable	4	56	60
	6	66	72

Figure 1. Breakdown of widowed sample from Study 1 according to Bugen's key concepts.

age. In both cases their husbands had died from arteriosclerotic heart disease and had not been ill.

The four subjects who identified the relationship as central and the death as not preventable were widows. The widows ranged in age from 49 to 63 years ($M = 57.3$ years). The deceased husbands' causes of death included a myocardial infarction, an aneurysm (history of chronic obstructive lung disease), and cancer. The length of time ill ranged from 0 to 66 months ($M = 19.3$).

The majority of subjects (91.7%) identified the relationship as peripheral. Of these 66 subjects, 7 widows and 3 widowers identified the death as preventable. The mean age of the 10 subjects was 62.4 years (range 43 to 78). The length of the deceased spouse's illness ranged from 0 to 60 months ($M = 19.0$). Of the 10 deceased spouses 5 had died from cancer. The remaining spouses had died from an aneurysm, a cerebral hemorrhage, complications from diabetes, and myocardial infarctions.

The remaining 56 subjects identified the relationship as peripheral and the death as not preventable. The mean age of the 36 widows and 20 widowers was 64.9 years (range 24 to 83). The mean time the deceased spouses had been ill was 30.4 months (range of 0 to 252). The causes of death included: 29 cancer victims, 19 heart-related deaths, a cerebral vascular accident, complications from diabetes, lung-related diseases, and renal failure.

Question 1. Are there differences in the grief experience for those who perceived the relationship as central and those who perceived the relationship as peripheral? For the measures of grief, those subjects who perceived the relationship as central experienced a greater Atypical Response, Anger/Hostility, Rumination, Somatization, and Loss of Appetite. Results are presented in Table 1. Note that only on the scales of Anger/Hostility and Somatization is the assumption of homogeneity of variance met.

Question 2. Are there differences in the grief experience between those who perceive the deceased's death as preventable and those who perceive the death as unpreventable? Those surviving spouses who perceived that their spouse's death was preventable experienced significantly more guilt ($F(1,71) = 9.27, p = .003$) than those who felt the death was not preventable. Mean guilt scores were 2.50 and 1.08 respectively. The Bartlett-Box F test was not significant ($F = 1.98, p = .16$).

In summary, even though a regression approach analysis of variance and tests for homogeneity of variance were utilized, results can only be considered suggestive. The low response rate further limits the ability to generalize from the findings. Consequently, the need for additional qualitative research with the concepts was identified in order to explore the complexity of the concepts, as well as to address measurement concerns that arose.

STUDY 2

An exploratory, descriptive design using qualitative and quantitative methods was used in Study 2. The purpose was to describe Bugen's concepts of centrality and preventability using semi-structured short answer questions.

Methods and Sample

A letter describing the research was sent to all active caregivers and randomly selected bereaved caregivers who met the criteria for inclusion during 1985-1986. A member of the research team then contacted the caregiver by phone to answer any questions and determine the person's willingness to participate in the one-time face-to-face interview. Thirty-two active caregivers and 32 bereaved caregivers were sent letters about the research. Twenty active and 20 bereaved caregivers agreed to participate resulting in a response rate of 63%. An additional three active caregivers were sent information; however, the care receivers died prior to the follow-up call.

TABLE 1. Significant ANOVAs for Study 1 Subjects' Perception of Relationship as Central or Peripheral

Main Effect	Central		Peripheral			
	Mean	St.Dev.	Mean	St.Dev.	F	Bartlett p
Atypical Response	9.00	5.29	4.95	2.30	13.00**	9.83 .002
Anger/Hostility	5.17	2.93	2.82	1.88	7.79*	2.21 .138
Rumination	7.33	3.67	4.41	2.01	10.00*	4.52 .034
Somatization	10.17	4.02	5.00	3.11	14.50**	.67 .414
Loss Appetite	2.33	1.86	.79	1.02	10.90*	4.57 .030

Note dfs = 1,71.

*p < .01

**p < .001

The majority of subjects were interviewed in their homes by one of two interviewers trained in the use of the interview guides. The interviews were audiotaped and the interviewer recorded the subject's responses. The handwritten responses were transcribed and verified with the audiotape for accuracy and completeness. The qualitative data was analyzed using the Ethnograph software package (Siedel, Kjolseth & Clark, 1985). The Ethnograph allows the researcher to organize the data on a personal computer and to label segments of data into meaningful pieces for retrieval purposes.

The study was undertaken with 20 family members who were currently caring for a terminally ill spouse or parent (active caregiver) and 20 family members who had cared for a terminally ill spouse or parent (bereaved caregivers). All of the caregivers had, or were, receiving services through a home-based hospice program in the Pacific Northwest. Criteria for inclusion in the study for both the active and bereaved caregivers included the following: the caregiver was either a spouse caring for a terminally ill spouse or an adult child caring for a terminally ill parent, the care receiver was 40 years of age or older, and the family had been admitted to the program for at least two weeks. An additional criteria for the bereaved caregivers was that the death had occurred within the past 12 months.

Interview Guide

Interview guides for the active and bereaved caregivers were developed and pretested for clarity of questions. The relationship between the caregivers and care receivers, or centrality, was explored in relation to four domains. The domains were identified through a review of existing literature on adult relationships and clinical practice. They included: (1) feelings of respect for the care receiver, (2) the love shared between the caregiver and care receiver, (3) how much the caregiver depended on the care receiver for daily activities or tasks, and (4) the caregiver questioning how, or even whether, he/she would survive without the ill person in his/her life.

The subjects were asked to describe their perception of the specific domain and then they were asked to rate the domain on a scale of 1 to 10, with 1 representing a minimal score and 10 representing a great deal. For example, bereaved caregivers were asked the following in relation to love shared:

> Family members also think about how the deceased person did, or did not make them feel loved. Some family members feel that the person offered them a great deal of love and nurturance while others feel that the person offered them minimal love or support. As you think about the love and nurturance shared between (CARE RECEIVER'S NAME) and you, how would you describe it? . . . On a scale of 1 to 10, with 1 representing minimal love and nurturance and 10 representing a great deal of love and nurturance, how would you rate the love and nurturance shared between (CARE RECEIVER'S NAME) and you?

Subjects were also asked whether their feelings of respect and love had changed since the care receiver had become ill.

The active and bereaved caregivers' perception of preventability of the illness was measured on a 10-point scale with 1 representing absolutely not preventable and 10 absolutely preventable. The bereaved caregivers were also asked to rate their perception of the preventability of the care receiver's death using a similar scale. Although Bugen (1979) did not specify whether preventability was in relation to the death or the illness, a number of the widows and widowers interviewed in 1984 raised this question.

Findings

Demographic information is presented followed by the findings for Bugen's concepts of preventability and centrality. Demographic information on the active and bereaved caregivers and care receivers is provided in Table 2. It is interesting to note that there was a great deal of variability in the reference points used by the caregivers for specifying the length of the care receiver's illness. For example, some caregivers cited the time since the diagnosis was first made and others cited the time since the care receiver's condition worsened (e.g., became wheelchair-bound and gave up) as the start of the care receiver's illness.

The active caregivers included three wives, six husbands, eight daughters, and three sons. The nine spouses had been married an

TABLE 2. Demographic Information on Study 2 Caregivers and Care Receivers

	Mean	Range
Active Cases		
Caregiver Age in Years	55.5	25-78
Care Receiver Characteristics: Age in Years	69.5	53-95
Weeks between Hospice Admission and Interview	13.9	2-53
Months Ill	20.8	1-72
Bereaved Cases		
Caregiver Characteristics: Age in Years	60.6	23-84
Weeks since Death	23.3	8-52
Deceased Care Receiver Characteristics: Age in Years	70.4	45-94
Weeks from Hospice Admission to Death	7.0	1-17
Months Ill	15.2	3-60

average of 40.8 years, with this being the first marriage in 67% of the cases. The majority of active care receivers ($n = 17$) had been diagnosed with cancer. The remaining diagnoses included congestive heart failure, chronic obstructive pulmonary disease, and hepatic liver disease.

The bereaved caregivers included thirteen wives, two husbands, four daughters and one son. The fifteen spouses had been married an average of 38.2 years, with 80% of these marriages being the first one. All of the deceased care receivers had been diagnosed with cancer.

Centrality

Quantitative data on three of the four measures of centrality are provided in Table 3. The four domains of centrality measured included respect, love shared, dependency and survival.

The active caregivers expressed a great deal of respect for the care receiver ($M = 9.0$), however two children did rate their respect as a 4 or 5. The one child expressed "there is more duty than love involved" and the other described her parent's prejudices and how that had affected her life. Half of the active caregivers identified their respect as being the same, 45% identified their respect as having increased, and one person expressed that it had decreased.

Selected comments from the ten caregivers who experienced an increase in their respect for the care receiver include: "Because of her condition I give her a lot more consideration than before when she was able to handle things on her own," "She has never been easy to get along with . . . somehow, either she's changed or I have, now it is easy to live with her," "Her faith and her character, she is still a strong person and has her serenity," and "Just the fact that she is ill." The one person who identified a decrease in respect stated "He's not the same person . . . he is touchy and sometimes I feel that he is milking me for all I'm worth."

The bereaved caregivers also rated their respect for the deceased care receivers as a great deal ($M = 9.0$). Again, half of the caregivers felt that their feelings of respect for the care receiver had increased. Their comments included "I gained an appreciation of what he really was," "he never complained, he was a very fine man and he stayed that way," and "she displayed courage and a

TABLE 3. Quantitative Measures of Centrality and Preventability from Study 2

	Mean	SD	Range	n
Active Caregivers				
Centrality				
Feelings of Respect	9.00	1.78	4-10	18
Love Shared	8.76	2.22	3-10	17
Dependence for Daily Activities/Tasks	5.44	3.98	1-10	16
Preventability				
Illness	2.71	1.93	1-5	17
Bereaved Caregivers				
Centrality				
Feelings of Respect	9.00	1.49	5-10	20
Love Shared	8.31	2.09	4-10	18
Dependence for Daily Activities/Tasks	6.68	3.20	1-10	17
Preventability				
Illness	3.20	2.02	1-6	15
Death	2.16	2.29	1-9	16

positive approach throughout her illness." None of the bereaved caregivers felt that their respect had decreased. The three subjects, two children and one spouse, who rated their respect as 5, 6 or 7 shared comments that reflected ambivalence about the relationship and the sense that the care receiver was not a positive role model.

The love shared between the caregiver and care receiver was also measured. The mean score of 8.76 for the active caregivers represents a great deal of love, however the range in scores of 3-10 reflects divergent experiences. The two children who rated their respect for the care receiver as low also rated their love shared as low. A third person, a spouse who rated the love shared as a 5, expressed the following: "He is completely and totally self-centered at this time . . . everything for him has to come first regardless of how it affects the family . . . maybe he can't help it but this is going to destroy all of us." This woman also expressed that the love shared had decreased.

Half of the caregivers said that the love shared was the same, seven said it had increased and two chose not to respond. Examples of the comments for those caregivers who experienced an increase include: "The situation is different now, we're living together and she has me all to herself . . . that is something she has wanted all the years that I was married," "It has increased because we're under each other's feet all the time," and "Just to see someone that is ill and you can't help them . . . you feel so sorry."

The bereaved caregiver's perception of the love shared between him/her and the care receiver was also explored ($M = 8.31$) and the responses varied (range 4-10). Again, half of the subjects indicated that the feelings of love had increased since the care receiver had become ill. Examples of their comments included: "You know that you're going to lose that person and you can't see life without him, what you want to do is hold on to him," "we had a closeness and were able to spend time together," "there was a greater openness in the relationship," and "I never really knew him before he was ill." One subject indicated that the love had decreased due to the care receiver's response: "after she got sick she was taking drugs and she got down . . . she became negative and there was nothing I could do right, she hated me."

The third domain that the bereaved caregivers were asked about was the dependence between the caregiver and care receiver to daily activities and tasks. The mean dependency score for the active care-givers was 5.44, with a range of 1-10. Four active caregivers did not rate their dependency. Examples of their comments include "I didn't depend on him, I expected it" and "I depended on him and him on me."

Overall, the bereaved caregivers rated their dependency as moderate, or 6.68. However, there were two subjects who rated their dependency as a 1 or 2, or minimal, and four subjects who rated their dependency as a 10, or a great deal.

The last area that the caregivers were asked about is whether they questioned their own survival. Two active caregivers did not answer the question directly, 75% (n = 15) responded no, and 20% (n = 4) responded yes. The two caregivers who did not use the response set stated: "It's going to be lonely and the house will be empty . . . it's going to be tough . . . they say time is a healer, I hope it is" and "I'm not sure how to answer, I know I'll survive but it'll be hard not having her around." All but two of the bereaved caregivers had not questioned their own survival.

Preventability

The findings on the quantitative measures of preventability are provided in Table 3. Both active and bereaved caregivers were asked about the preventability of the care receiver's illness. The bereaved caregivers were also asked about the preventability of the death.

Overall, the active caregivers did not perceive the care receiver's illness as preventable (M = 2.71). However, six of the caregivers did select the middle point, or a score of 5, when they were asked about preventability. Selected comments from these caregivers included:

The specialist attributed his illness to smoking.

She had cancer a long time ago. She'd been keeping up and everything was negative so she didn't go in for checkups.

I suspect that it could have been discovered earlier, whether that makes it preventable is debatable.

It was colon cancer and he had poor bowel habits. He was also a heavy smoker and an intense person. There is cancer in his family. He had always gotten physicals but screening for colon cancer wasn't included.

Quite a few doctors have examined her and haven't concluded what the original source was.

I think the emphysema may have been prevented if he had stopped smoking years ago.

The bereaved caregivers also perceived the deceased care receiver's illness and death as not preventable ($M = 3.20$). However, seven of the subjects did rate the illness preventability as a 5 or 6. Examples of their comments included:

I just don't know, if I had realized sooner, his body was always so warm.

I always felt, I didn't tell her this, that she took too much medicine and I think that helped bring it on.

His illness might have been prevented if he would have changed his diet in earlier times, if he had cut out fats.

He smoked a great deal early, but he hadn't for 15-20 years. The smoking probably had something to do with it . . . If he had been going to a different doctor and had chest x-rays it might have been prevented . . . They are finding that a lot of these cancers are preventable, aren't they?

They say it wasn't related to her smoking, she smoked all her life. Medically, I think if they had gotten to it sooner they may have been able to treat it. Healthwise, if her attitude had been better.

Yes, I would think if he hadn't smoked, drank alcohol, and been a heavy coffee drinker. It happened over a long period of time. At least the doctor said that those three things in excess could have caused it. I guess it could have been preventable but the cure would have had to start a long time ago.

The comments of the five subjects who did not rate whether the illness was preventable tended to express that it was not preventable or that they were ambivalent. For example, "I don't see how it could be . . . it just got in there and grew . . . I don't think his smoking had anything to do with it" and "If he'd gone to the doctor sooner, maybe . . . I don't know with cancer you can't do anything with it."

The bereaved caregivers were also asked about the preventability of the death. The mean of 2.16 represents a general belief that the care receiver's death could not have been prevented; however, the range of scores from 1 to 9 represents divergent beliefs about preventability of the deaths. The three subjects who rated the preventability of the death as a 5 or greater referred back to the illness and whether it was preventable. For example, one caregiver stated "perhaps if he had not smoked then he wouldn't have had cancer, I think he could still be here." In addition, two subjects who did not rate the preventability of the death expressed that the question seemed the same as the one about illness preventability.

The other bereaved caregivers, who rated preventability from 1 to 4, tended to separate out whether the death was preventable. Some of their comments included: "Not after we found out about it, it was too late"; "No way, I've thought about that so many times and we did everything we could"; and, "It couldn't have been, they said there was nothing they could do."

In summary, 20 active and 20 bereaved caregivers described their relationship with the care receivers on four domains. The domains included respect, love shared, dependency and survival. The caregivers' responses tended to reflect the positiveness of the relationship; however, some caregivers did not use the rating scale. The caregivers also described and rated their perception of the preventability of the illness and death. The caregivers typically viewed the illness and death as not preventable. Again, some subjects did not use the rating scale. The small sample size is the major limitation of the study.

DISCUSSION

Implications for future research will be discussed since the purpose of Study 2 was to address measurement issues that arose from the Study 1 with the recently widowed. Additional methodological research needs to be undertaken with Bugen's concepts.

Two approaches to quantitatively measure centrality and preventability have been utilized, including forced choice items and Likert scales. The findings from the 1984 study, which utilized forced choice items, provided initial support for Bugen's concepts. However, two issues emerged from this work. First, the complexity of centrality, or the caregiver and care receiver relationship, needed to be expanded to include feelings of respect, the love shared, perceived dependency and questioning of survival. Second, for bereaved caregivers the issue of preventability needed to be explored in relation to the illness as well as the actual death.

The use of Likert scales in the more recent study yielded some interesting results. The caregivers' responses on the various scales did yield some variability, or range of scores, which is a positive finding. In comparison, Murphy (Chenell, 1986) utilized a 9-point Likert scale to measure centrality of the relationship for persons who had experienced a confirmed or presumed death from the Mt. St. Helen's eruption in 1980. All of the subjects ($N = 69$) rated the closeness of their relationship with the deceased as a 7 or greater (1 represented not at all close and 9 represented very close) which Murphy operationally defined as central relationships. The variability in the recent study may be due, in part, to the measurement of more specific domains of centrality versus a global measure like the one used by Murphy (1982).

Another finding involves missing data on the Likert scales. With the exception of the bereaved caregivers' rating on respect, from two to five subjects did not rate specific scales despite the fact that they were asked for a specific rating. Potential reasons for this missing data, based on the qualitative responses, are that the caregivers were ambivalent or unable to attach a number to their responses. One strategy for dealing with missing data would be to assign scores according to preestablished guidelines. This strategy was used in Study 1 when subjects were not willing to select one of the forced choice items. An alternative strategy would be to try an alternative rating scale, such as marking a response on a line with two anchors—very little or a great deal, which might reduce the frequency of missing data. Given the potential that caregivers will perceive information about the relationship as sensitive and/or private there may not be a simple solution that yields a 100% response.

An additional area that needs to be considered with the centrality of the relationship is the caregiver's satisfaction with the relationship. This issue emerged from the analysis of the quantitative and qualitative data across the various domains and in relation to current versus past feelings. There were a few caregivers who identified that they had very little to moderate feelings of love and respect for the care receiver. According to the Bugen's model one could predict that their grief would be mild since the relationship would appear to be peripheral. However, the caregiver's perception of the meaning of their feelings, or their satisfaction with any given area of the relationship, should be measured. For example, this could include whether there had been a decrease in feelings of respect, which was the case for one caregiver who described how her husband had become self-centered since becoming ill. Irrelevant of whether this caregiver rated her respect as low (peripheral) or high (central) she may feel guilty about her feelings of respect for her husband during her grief. The addition of a question to measure satisfaction with respect, love shared and dependency needs to be given additional consideration.

It is premature to say whether the inclusion of the four measures of centrality will yield greater predictive power when determining individuals at risk for prolonged or abnormal grief. However, this researcher is encouraged by the findings and will continue methodological work on the four domains.

Future research with Bugen's concepts should include the differentiation of whether the illness and/or death was believed to be preventable by bereaved caregivers. Despite the finding that some bereaved caregivers view the illness and death as one and the same, others did differentiate between the two. An additional area that needs to be systematically studied is who the caregiver perceives as responsible for preventing the illness and/or death. Some of the caregivers identified the care receiver as the one who was responsible (e.g., if he had quit smoking years ago or if she had not taken so many medications), while others viewed it as their responsibility (e.g., if I had noticed that he was so warm). The use of scales for measuring preventability of the illness and death would mask the subjects' underlying beliefs about who is responsible. At least, the subject should be asked to explain their rating.

Potential areas for future research include assessing bereaved individuals at various intervals during their grief experience in order to determine whether their perceptions about the relationship and preventability of the illness and death change. Although it was not the intent of the more recent study to compare the active and bereaved caregivers' responses the similarity of responses should be noted. Repeated measures of the concepts are needed in order to determine what, if any, changes occur with time.

Intervention strategies also need to be systematically developed and evaluated, with attention being given to Bugen's key concepts. Lastly, sample sizes need to be increased in hopes of including more subjects who identify with the central relationship statements. In order to undertake rigorous empirical research, the group sizes need to be similar and additional statistical controls need to be used.

CONCLUSION

Although the findings are limited by unequal group sizes, small sample sizes, and ongoing issues around measurement, there is evidence that Bugen's concepts of central/peripheral and preventable/not preventable are significant variables in the experience of grief. The work of Bugen was originally proposed as a model of prediction and intervention. Based on the findings from the two studies, it would be premature to significantly alter clinical practice based solely on the model. Clearly, additional systematic research is needed on measurement of the concepts and eventually systematic evaluation of the model in terms of prediction and intervention should be undertaken.

REFERENCES

Abrams, R.D. (1974). *Not alone with cancer*. Chicago: Charles C Thomas.

Bugen, L.A. (1979). *Death and dying theory/research/practice*. Dubuque, IA: William C. Brown.

Chenell, S.L. (1986). *Beliefs of preventability and unpreventability regarding circumstances of death in a disease bereaved sample*. Unpublished master's research project, The Oregon Health Sciences University School of Nursing, Portland, OR.

Clayton, P.J. (1979). The sequelae and nonsequelae of conjugal bereavement. *American Journal of Psychiatry, 101*, 141-148.

Gerber, I., rusalem, R., Hannon, N., Battin, D., & Arkin, A. (1975). Anticipatory grief and aged widows and widowers. *Journal of Gerontology, 30*, 225-229.

Kirschling, J.M. (1984). *Social support and coping in the recently widowed*. Unpublished doctoral dissertation, Indiana University School of Nursing, Indianapolis, IN.

Kirschling, J.M. (1986). The experience of terminal illness of adult family members. *The Hospice Journal, 2*(1), 121-138.

Murphy, S.A. (1982). Coping with stress following a natural disaster: The volcanic eruption of Mt. St. Helen's. *Dissertation Abstracts International, 42*, 10B, p. 4014. (University microfilm no. 82-07, 736).

Murphy, S.A. (1983). Theoretical perspectives on bereavement. In P.L. Chin (Ed.), *Advances in nursing theory development* (pp. 191-206). Rockville, MD: Aspen.

Olson, J.G. (1985). *The functional level of parents who experience a sudden and unexpected infant death 13 to 18 months after the event*. Unpublished master's thesis. The Oregon Health Sciences University School of Nursing, Portland, OR.

Osterweis, M., & Green, M. (Eds.) (1984). *Bereavement reactions, consequences, and care*. Washington, D.C.: National Academy Press.

Parkes, C.M., & Brown, R.J. (1972). Health after bereavement: A controlled study of young Boston widows and widowers. *Psychosomatic Medicine, 34*, 449-461.

Parkes, C.M., & Weiss, R.S. (1983). *Recovery from bereavement*. New York: Basic Books.

Sanders, C.M., Mauger, P.A., & Strong, P.N. (1979). *A manual for the grief experience inventory*. (Available from Catherine M. Sanders, Department Psychology, Sacred Heart College, Belmont, NC).

Siedel, J.V., Kjolseth, R., & Clark, J.A. (1985). *The ethnograph: A user's guide*. Littleton, CO: Qualia Research Associates.

Vachon, M. (1979, September). *The importance of social support in the longitudinal adaptation to bereavement and breast cancer*. Paper presented at the meeting of the American Psychological Association, New York.

Vachon, M.L.S., Sheldon, A.R., Lancee, W.J., Lyall, W.A.L., Rogers, J., & Freeman, S.J.J. (1982). Correlates of enduring distress patterns following bereavement: Social network, life situation and personality. *Psychological Medicine, 12*, 783-788.

Differentiating Grief and Depression

Paul J. Robinson
Stephen Fleming

SUMMARY. The present paper offers a selective review of the relevant empirical literature that has attempted to outline the reaction of a person to the death of a spouse, and the manner in which this reaction differs from a clinically significant depressive disorder. This review indicates that although grief and depression may be similar in some ways (e.g., affective and behavioural disruption), they rarely are similar in terms of level of pathology in cognitive functioning. In light of this, it is recommended that caregivers working with the bereaved go beyond assessment of depressive symptomatology, and explore the personal meaning of the death for the grieving spouse.

The present paper offers a selective review of the relevant empirical literature that has attempted to outline the typical reaction of a person to the death of a spouse, and the manner in which this reaction differs from a clinically significant depressive disorder.

According to the American Psychiatric Association's Diagnostic and Statistical Manual of Mental Disorders (DSM III-R, 1987), the category of "Uncomplicated Bereavement" (which is classified as a "V" Code, or a condition that is not attributed to a mental disorder) can be utilized by the diagnostician when the focus of attention or treatment is the normal reaction to the death of a loved one. This normal reaction is thought to be very similar to a full depressive syndrome, although the morbid preoccupation with personal worthlessness, prolonged and marked functional impairment, and marked psychomotor retardation typically identifiable in the person suffer-

Paul J. Robinson, PhD, is a psychologist at North York General Hospital, Psychology Dept., 4001 Leslie St., Willowdale, Ontario, Canada M2K 1E1. Stephen Fleming, PhD, is a psychologist in private practice, and Professor of Psychology at Atkinson College, York University, 4700 Keele St., North York, Ontario, Canada M3J 2R7.

77

ing from a clinically significant depressive disorder are thought to be uncommon. If these symptoms are present, it is argued that the bereavement reaction has been complicated by the development of a major depressive disorder.

The present delineation of uncomplicated bereavement as a discrete and identifiable phenomenon, separate from a major depression, was introduced in the 1980 version of the DSM (DSM III). In the version before that (DSM II 1968), it was not clear how the reaction to the death of a loved one was to be classified, if it was to be classified at all.

In spite of the more recent inclusion in DSM III of a separate category for an uncomplicated bereavement reaction, the discussion remains brief and descriptive, and does not seem to fully reflect the extent to which bereavement reactions have been investigated and discussed by modern researchers and writers. For example, numerous investigators and clinicians have concluded that there are bereavement reactions that may be considered as complicated, abnormal, or pathological, which are distinguishable from both uncomplicated bereavement and major depression (e.g., Briscoe & Smith, 1975; Demi & Miles, 1987; Robinson & Fleming, 1988; Schneider, 1980; Volkan, 1970; Worden, 1982). As noted by Hoagland (1984), however, the DSM III system clearly indicates that complicated bereavement does not exist, and the clinician or researcher is required to diagnose a complicated grief response as a depressive episode or as some other DSM III psychiatric disorder. If restricted to such a procedure, misdiagnosis appears to be a distinct possibility and, in turn, the chances of the implementation of an inappropriate and possibly harmful therapeutic intervention would seem to be increased. For example, antidepressant medication could be prescribed for an individual who is not experiencing a major depressive episode but, rather, who is experiencing a depressive-like, complicated reaction to a loss. It is not at all clear that this would be the treatment of choice in such a case.

SELECTIVE REVIEW
OF THE RELEVANT EMPIRICAL LITERATURE

In his classic paper, *Mourning and Melancholia*, Freud (1917/ 1957) observes that although grief and depression have a similar clinical picture, the negative self-regard often present in depression differentiates depression from normal sadness or grief. It was not until Lindemann's 1944 investigation of the survivors of the Coconut Grove fire, however, that bereavement was recognized as a subject worthy of systematic investigation. As Fulton (1970) and Kastenbaum and Costa (1977) point out, research still did not burgeon until the appearance of Herman Feifel's book, *The Meaning of Death*, in 1959. Since that publication, a myriad of theoretical-conceptual discussions and empirical investigations has emerged. Although this development may be desirable, the rate and volume of work seems to have contributed to a confusion of conjecture and postulation with data-based information. In the following selective review, therefore, an attempt is made to isolate the relevant empirical literature, and to identify features of grief and depression that have emerged from such systematic investigations.

Researchers have drawn conclusions about the similarities and differences between grief and depression based on various types of comparisons of bereaved and nonbereaved individuals. For example, while some researchers have drawn conclusions based on the study of bereaved subjects only (e.g., Clayton et al., 1968), others have compared depressed bereaved subjects to depressed nonbereaved subjects (e.g., Briscoe & Smith, 1975). Studies representative of these designs are outlined Table 1.

As indicated by Table 1, there is a progression of comparisons ranging from the study of bereaved subjects only, to the inclusion of nonbereaved control subjects, to the differentiation of bereaved subjects (or uncomplicated bereaved) from bereaved depressives (or complicated bereaved), to the comparison of bereaved subjects with nonbereaved depressives, and finally to the comparison of bereaved depressives with nonbereaved depressives. It is noteworthy that there is a substantial decline in the number of studies as the comparison of bereavement reactions with depression becomes increasingly obvious and direct.

With regard to the question of differentiating uncomplicated bereavement from depression, those studies that have investigated bereaved subjects only, or bereaved vs. nonbereaved control subjects, are of limited value. In general, the findings seem to indicate that up to the end of the first year of bereavement, the symptomatology of grief may be similar to a clinical depression. Specifically,

Table 1

Representative Comparisons in the Bereavement Literature*

	Bereaved	Bereaved Depressed	Nonbereaved Depressed
Controls	Carey 1977 Gallagher et. al. 1982 Maddison & Viola 1968 Parkes & Brown 1972 Sanders 1979-80, 1980-81 Vachon et. al. 1976		
Bereaved	Ball 1976-77 Barrett & Schneweiss 1980 Blanchard et. al. 1976 Clayton et. al. 1968 Goddard & Leviton 1973 Hardt 1978 Heyman & Gianturco 1973 Lindemann 1944 Marris 1958 Parkes 1972, 1975 Pennebaker & O'Heeron 1984 Sheskin & Wallace 1976 Vargas et. al. 1984	Bornstein & Clayton 1972 Bornstein et. al. 1973 Clayton et. al. 1972 Parkes 1965a Parkes 1965b Robinson & Fleming 1988	Clayton et. al. 1974 Gallagher et. al. 1982 Robinson & Fleming 1988
Bereaved Depressed		Abrahms 1981 Horowitz et. al. 1980	Briscoe & Smith 1975 Robinson & Fleming 1988

* When there is an intersection of a row and a column with the same heading (e.g., both row and column are headed "Bereaved"), this means that only this group was considered in the study (e.g., bereaved subjects only).

many authors have noted appetite disturbances, sleep disturbances, dysphoria, fatigue, and loss of interest in previously pleasurable activities as being involved in the typical reaction to bereavement (Blanchard, Blanchard, & Becker, 1976; Carey, 1977; Clayton, Desmarais, & Winokur, 1968; Lindemann, 1944; Maddison & Viola, 1968; Marris, 1958; Parkes, 1972, 1975; Parkes & Brown, 1972; Sanders, 1979-80, 1980-81). All of these symptoms are noted as criteria for a major depressive episode (DSM III-R, 1987).

What appears to be lacking in the uncomplicated or typical grief reaction, however, are the supposedly unique self-centered cognitive features of depression. Consistent with Freud's (1917/1957) conceptualization of mourning (i.e., uncomplicated bereavement), Clayton et al. (1968), Lindemann (1944), and Parkes (1972, 1975) all have noted a lack of the persistent self-condemnation, suicidal ideation, and general negative self-perceptions that may be involved in a clinically significant depression (Beck, Rush, Shaw, & Emery, 1979; DSM III-R, 1987).

Thus, based on these studies of bereaved subjects only, and of bereaved vs. control subjects, it appears that grief is most similar to depression in terms of affect and behaviour (e.g., dysphoric mood, physical effects, withdrawal from social situations), and most dissimilar in terms of cognition. The lack of a depressed comparison group in these investigations, however, makes it inappropriate to draw any firm conclusions.

In an effort to counteract this problem and gain further insight into possible distinguishing features, several investigators have attempted to compare nondepressed bereaved subjects with other bereaved subjects who have been classified as depressed.

These investigations of nondepressed and depressed bereaved have indicated that the symptomatology found within groups of bereaved individuals who also have been classified as depressed has generally been very similar, in kind, to the symptomatology found in the typical, expected reaction to loss (Abrahms, 1981; Bornstein & Clayton, 1972; Bornstein, Clayton, Halikas, Maurice, & Robins, 1973; Clayton, Halikas, & Maurice, 1972; Horowitz, Wilner, Marmar, & Krupnick, 1980; Parkes, 1965a). Consistent with the findings of those studies that have investigated bereaved subjects only, and with those that have utilized a nonbereaved control group for purposes of comparison, it is found that the typical grief reaction is indistinguishable in many ways from those reactions that also involve more depressive-like features. The results of those studies in which nondepressed bereaved have been compared with depressed bereaved have further indicated, however, that this common symptomatology may be much more intense and persistent within the depressed bereaved than within the nondepressed bereaved.

The role of cognitive factors in the differentiation of uncomplicated and complicated reactions to loss also is evident from the research that has considered depressed and nondepressed outcomes following bereavement. The systematic and clinical research of Parkes (1965a), Clayton et al. 1972), Horowitz et al. (1980), and Abrahms (1981), in particular, has indicated that a depressive-like reaction to bereavement is more likely to be accompanied by thoughts of hopelessness, self-blame, and guilt than is a nondepressed reaction.

Although such a cognitive pattern seems similar to that expected for a clinical depression, the lack of a nonbereaved depressed comparison group makes it difficult to draw conclusions about the depression of widowhood as compared with major depressive disorder unrelated to bereavement. Nevertheless, Clayton and her colleagues have argued that the depression of widowhood is different from other types of depression in several ways. Specifically, these authors have pointed to the equal numbers of men and women, the lack of a significantly greater number of first-degree relatives who have suffered from a clinical depression, and the lack of a personal history of clinical depression within those groups of bereaved who have also been classified as depressed.

The research reviewed to this point has indicated that although the typical reaction to loss may be similar in many ways to a clinical depression, there appear to be significant differences (e.g., the lack of negative, self-centred cognitions in the typical reaction). Moreover, there may be atypical, complicated reactions to loss that differ from both the uncomplicated, typical reaction to bereavement (e.g., the complicated manifest a more intense and persistent depressive symptomatology), and from a major depressive disorder (e.g., although in general more women than men receive the diagnosis of depression, this sex difference is not found in the depressed bereaved). Unfortunately, the relationship among these three potential outcomes (i.e., uncomplicated, complicated, and depressed) remains uncertain because of the lack of comparisons to nonbereaved, clinically diagnosed depressives. In an effort to counteract this problem, a few investigators have directly compared various groups of bereaved individuals to groups of nonbereaved depressed individuals.

Briscoe and Smith (1975), Clayton, Herjanic, Murphy, and Woodruff (1974), and Gallagher, Dessonville, Breckenridge, Thompson, and Amaral (1982) utilized nonbereaved depressive groups for purposes of comparison to bereaved subjects. The results of these investigations corroborate the conclusions of the already mentioned research in which no nonbereaved depressed comparison group was included. That is, there appear to be bereavement reactions that may be subclassified as uncomplicated and complicated (i.e., depressive-like), neither of which is tantamount to a clinical depression. Gallagher et al. (1982) was the only investigation in this group of studies that directly and systematically considered the role of cognitive factors in the differentiation of grief and depression. These authors found a sample of recently widowed elderly (uncomplicated in their bereavement) to be significantly less likely to endorse self-deprecatory items on a measure of depressive symptomatology (i.e., the Beck Depression Inventory, Beck, Ward, Mendelson, Mock, & Erbaugh, 1961) than were a comparable sample of nonbereaved depressives.

Consistent with the conclusions of Gallagher et al., Robinson and Fleming (1988) recently found significantly less cognitive dysfunction in middle-aged bereaved widows compared to nonbereaved psychiatric depressives. Unlike Gallagher et al., however, Robinson and Fleming utilized instruments specifically designed to measure cognitive functioning and, moreover, included a group of bereaved subjects who met the DSM III criteria for a major depression (i.e., complicated bereaved). In spite of receiving the same interview-determined diagnosis as the psychiatric depressed, this group of complicated bereaved did not at all manifest the high level of cognitive dysfunction that was manifested in the psychiatric depressed. In agreement with Clayton and her colleagues, Robinson and Fleming concluded that the depression of widowhood was not tantamount to depression unrelated to bereavement.

CONCLUSION

In the American Psychiatric Association Diagnostic and Statistical Manual of Mental Disorders (DSM III-R, 1987), a distinction is made between uncomplicated bereavement and major depressive disorder. A survey of the empirical literature appears to support such a distinction, although there is clear overlap in symptomatology between these two phenomena, especially when those early in their grief are considered. In spite of these similarities between uncomplicated bereavement and clinical depression, however, several investigators have concluded that bereaved and depressed individuals rarely are similar in terms of cognition. By the use of research designs of varying degrees of assurance of validity, numerous researchers including Abrahms (1981), Bornstein et al. (1973), Clayton et al. (1974), Gallagher et al. (1982), Horowitz et al. (1980), Lindemann (1944), Parkes (1965a), and Robinson and Fleming (1988) all have pointed to the role of persistent, distorted, and negative perceptions of self, experience, and future in the differentiation of major depressive disorder from uncomplicated bereavement. These conclusions are consistent with the theoretical formulations of Freud (1917/1957).

Although the present consideration of the empirical literature appears to support this distinction made by DSM III-R with regard to uncomplicated bereavement and major depressive disorder, it also indicates the shortcomings of such a simple distinction. In contrast to the notions outlined in DSM III-R, many authors and researchers have discussed the possibility of the development of a complicated bereavement reaction. For example, Lindemann (1944) has referred to "morbid grief reactions," and Parkes (1965b) has referred to "variants of grief." The empirical work of Briscoe and Smith (1975) and Robinson and Fleming (1988), in particular, has indicated that there may be a distinct, depressive-like bereavement outcome separate from both an uncomplicated bereavement and a major depression.

In her 1983 discussion of the factors affecting the outcome of conjugal bereavement, Raphael observed that in the area of personality variables, no specific risk factors had been identified in the bereavement literature. The present review indicates that a worthwhile starting point in studying "personality factors" may be the area of cognitive style. As every caregiver of the bereaved already knows, the death of a spouse does not lead to identical reactions in the bereaved. Personal meaning of the loss is a powerful mediating influence in the grief reaction. Future research would do well to further investigate the role of this and other "personality" factors as they relate to bereavement outcome.

CLINICAL IMPLICATIONS

The present selective literature review indicates that when a caregiver encounters a bereaved individual, it is not adequate simply to investigate the criteria for a major depression. The depression of widowhood is not tantamount to a psychiatric depression, even when the criteria for a major depressive episode have been met by the bereaved person. Although the complicated bereaved spouse may manifest a depressive symptomatology, this syndrome may be more similar to uncomplicated grief than it is to a clinical depression. In line with this conclusion, Worden (1982) states that there is

> more of a continuous relationship between normal and abnormal grief reactions, between the complicated and the uncomplicated, and that pathology is more related to the intensity of a reaction or the duration of a reaction rather than to the simple presence or absence of a specific behaviour. (p. 58)

With regard to the differentiation of bereavement reactions from major depression, attention to self-related cognitive processes seems to be of particular value. As Rando (1984) observed, too often when caregivers encounter a bereaved individual, the sole focus is on the individual's reactions to the external world, with relatively little attention paid to cognitive and intrapsychic processes. The present discussion seems to indicate the benefit of fully exploring with the bereaved person his or her view of self, world, and future, i.e., the personal meaning of the loss for that person. Such an exploration allows the caregiver to more accurately identify the nature of the bereavement reaction and, in turn, more appropriately and effectively intervene.

REFERENCES

Abrahms, J. (1981). Depression versus normal grief following the death of a significant other. In G. Emery, S. Hollon, & R. Bedrosian (Eds.), *New directions in cognitive therapy* (pp. 255-270). New York: Guilford Press.

American Psychiatric Association. (1968). *Diagnostic and statistical manual of mental disorders* (2nd ed.). Washington, D.C.: Author.

American Psychiatric Association. (1980). *Diagnostic and statistical manual of mental disorders* (3rd ed.). Washington, D.C.: Author.

American Psychiatric Association. (1987). *Diagnostic and statistical manual of mental disorders* (rev. 3rd ed.). Washington, D.C.: Author.

Ball, J. (1976-77). Widow's grief: The impact of age and mode of death. *Omega*, 7, 307-333.

Barrett, C., & Schneweis, K. (1980-81). An empirical search for stages of widowhood. *Omega, 11*, 97-104.

Beck, A., Rush, A., Shaw, B., & Emery, G. (1979). *Cognitive therapy of depression*. New York: Guilford Press.

Beck, A., Ward, C., Mendelson, M., Mock, J., & Erbaugh, J. (1961). An inventory for measuring depression. *Archives of General Psychiatry, 4*, 561-571.

Blanchard, C., Blanchard, E., & Becker, J. (1976). The young widow: Depressive symptomatology throughout the grief process. *Psychiatry, 39*, 394-399.

Bornstein, P., & Clayton, P. (1972). The anniversary reaction. *Diseases of the Nervous System, 33*, 470-472.

Bornstein, P., Clayton, P., Halikas, J., Maurice, W., & Robins, E. (1973). The depression of widowhood after thirteen months. *British Journal of Psychiatry, 122*, 561-566.

Briscoe, C., & Smith, J. (1975). Depression in bereavement and divorce. *Archives of General Psychiatry, 32*, 439-443.

Carey, R. (1977). The widowed: A year later. *Journal of Counseling Psychology, 24*, 125-131.

Clayton, P., Desmarais, L., & Winokur, G. (1968). A study of normal bereavement. *American Journal of Psychiatry, 125*, 168-178.

Clayton, P., Halikas, J., & Maurice, W. (1972). The depression of widowhood. *British Journal of Psychiatry, 120*, 71-78.

Clayton, P., Herjanic, M., Murphy, G., & Woodruff, R. (1974). Mourning and depression: Their similarities and differences. *Canadian Psychiatric Association Journal, 19*, 309-312.

Demi, A., & Miles, M. (1987). Parameters of normal grief: A Delphi study. *Death Studies, 11*, 397-412.

Freud, S. (1957). Mourning and melancholia. In J. Strachey (Ed. and Trans.), *The standard edition of the complete psychological works of Sigmund Freud* (Vol. 14, pp. 243-258). London: Hogarth Press. (Original work published 1917).

Fulton, R. (1970). Death, grief, and social recuperation. *Omega, 1*, 23-28.

Gallagher, D., Dessonville, C., Breckenridge, J., Thompson, L., & Amaral, P. (1982). Similarities and differences between normal grief and depression in older adults. *Essence, 5*, 127-140.

Goddard, H., & Leviton, D. (1980). Intimacy-sexual needs of the bereaved: An exploratory study. *Death Education, 3*, 347-358.

Hardt, D. (1978). An investigation of the stages of bereavement. *Omega, 9*, 279-285.

Heyman, D., & Gianturco, D. (1973). Long-term adaptation by the elderly to bereavement. *Journal of Gerontology, 28*, 359-362.

Hoagland, A. (1984). Bereavement and personal constructs: Old theories and new concepts. In F. Epting & R. Neimeyer (Eds.), *Personal meanings of death* (pp. 89-107). New York: Hemisphere/McGraw-Hill.

Horowitz, M., Wilner, N., Marmar, C., & Krupnick, J. (1980). Pathological grief and the activation of latent self-images. *American Journal of Psychiatry, 137*, 1157-1162.

Kastenbaum, R., & Costa, P. (1977). Psychological perspectives on death. *Annual Review of Psychology, 28*, 225-249.

Lindemann, E. (1944). Symptomatology and management of grief. *American Journal of Psychiatry, 101*, 141-148.

Maddison, D., & Viola, A. (1968). The health of widows in the year following bereavement. *Journal of Psychosomatic Research, 12*, 297-306.

Marris, P. (1958). *Widows and their families*. London: Routledge & Kegan Paul.

Parkes, C. (1965a). Bereavement and mental illness: Part 1 — A clinical study of the grief of bereaved psychiatric patients. *British Journal of Medical Psychology, 38*, 1-12.

Parkes, C. (1965b). Bereavement and mental illness: Part 2 — A classification of bereavement reactions. *British Journal of Medical Psychology, 38*, 13-26.

Parkes, C. (1972). *Bereavement: Studies of grief in adult life*. New York: International Universities Press.

Parkes, C. (1975). Determinants of outcome following bereavement. *Omega, 6*, 303-323.

Parkes, C., & Brown, R. (1972). Health after bereavement: A controlled study of young Boston widows and widowers. *Psychosomatic Medicine, 34*, 449-461.

Pennebaker, J., & O'Heeron, R. (1984). Confiding in others and illness rate among spouses of suicide and accidental-death victims. *Journal of Abnormal Psychology, 93,* 473-476.

Rando, T. (1984). *Grief, dying, and death: Clinical interventions for caregivers.* Champaign, IL: Research Press.

Raphael, B. (1983). *The anatomy of bereavement.* New York: Basic.

Robinson, P., & Fleming, S. (1988, June). *Depressotypic cognitive patterns in conjugal bereavement and major depression.* Paper presented at the Annual Meeting of the Canadian Psychological Association, Montreal, Quebec.

Sanders, C. (1979-80). Comparison of adult bereavement in the death of a spouse, child, and parent. *Omega, 10,* 303-322.

Sanders, C. (1980-81). Comparison of younger and older spouses in bereavement outcome. *Omega, 11,* 217-232.

Schneider, J. (4th Quarter, 1980). Clinically significant differences between grief, pathological grief, and depression. *Patient Counseling and Education,* 161-169.

Sheskin, A., & Wallace, S. (1976). Differing bereavements: Suicide, natural, and accidental death. *Omega, 7,* 229-242.

Vachon, M., Formo, A., Freedman, K., Lyall, W., Rogers, J., & Freeman, S. (1976). Stress reactions to bereavement. *Essence, 1,* 15-21.

Vargas, L., Loya, F., & Hodde-Vargas, J. (1984, August). *Grief across modes of death in three ethnic groups.* Paper presented at the 92nd Annual Convention of the American Psychological Association, Toronto, Ont., Canada.

Volkan, V. (1970). Typical findings in pathological grief. *Psychiatric Quarterly, 44,* 231-250.

Worden, J.W. (1982). *Grief counseling and grief therapy: A handbook for the mental health practitioner.* New York: Spring.

Grieving as a Hero's Journey

Bonnie Sigren Busick

SUMMARY. The psychodynamics of transformation through grief and loss can be explained through a model of personal growth which encompasses both the individuation process of Jungian psychology and the hero's journey which Joseph Campbell explored through mythology. The model may provide a tool for hospice caregivers to use in assessing both their own responses to death and dying and their grieving patients'/families' needs for assistance.

Along with their deep sense of tragedy, some bereaved persons also report that working through grief has led them to a period of intensified growth and understanding. As a result of this growth, their existence has become more meaningful and they have gained a deeper appreciation for the value of life, both their own and others.

Using evidence of this transformative experience, bereavement counselors have formulated models for the successful resolution of loss. The changes in attitudes and behaviors which accompany this model are easily identified, but the psychological processes which bring about these changes have not been well elucidated. Humanistic psychologies recognize transformation, but don't explain the psychodynamics of the process. On the other hand, transpersonal psychology focuses on the psychological events which characterize transformation and its theories may possibly provide a means for

Bonnie Sigren Busick, PhD, RN, a nurse and consultant with Boulder County Hospice for four years, is team trainer for Hospice of Boulder Memorial Hospital. She is adjunct faculty at Boulder Graduate School and Ernest Holmes School of Ministry. Author of *Ill Not Insane*, she is also a freelance lecturer, consultant and seminar leader. Address correspondence to the author c/o New Ideas Seminars, P.O. Box 13683, Boulder, CO 80308-3683.

more fully understanding the psychological challenges and pitfalls of grief.

One model for explaining the psychodynamics of transformation through grief is found by combining theories of the scholar Joseph Campbell, who extensively studied world mythology (Campbell, 1968), and psychologist Carl G. Jung (Jung, 1958 & 1971). Using the hero of mythology, Campbell sees personal growth represented by the stages of the hero's journey and Jung uses heroes to represent aspects of the psyche. Following their format, the hero's journey can be both a symbol and a model for the processes of transformation through grief.

The potential value of using the transpersonal model is twofold. First, it may provide hospice staff and volunteers with an effective method for examining their own relationships to grief. In other words, they can examine their own journeys by applying this psychological model to their attitudes and dreams, thereby helping them to grow as human beings as well as hospice caregivers. Patients/families, the unit of care for hospices, benefit both from the caregivers' personal knowledge of the journey and their understanding of the psychological theories behind it. As caregivers enhance their own personal awareness, they have a more comprehensive perspective from which to assess their grieving patients'/families' progress and to determine the most appropriate intervention.

Caregivers' transpersonal assessment of both themselves and their patients/families depends on knowledge of personal and transpersonal symbols, such as drowning and rescue images. These images represent the nonverbal language of the unconscious and may appear in dreams, fantasies and active imagination, the latter a Jungian technique for completing or expanding on information from dreams and fantasies (Jung, 1971). With information from these symbols, caregivers can help some patients/families understand the transpersonal nature of the grieving process and then guide them toward a resolution of the issues which surround their pain. For others, caregivers may find that the dreams of family members indicate that the bereaved are holding onto the past and have not integrated the death of their loved one.

This model of transformation through grief is based on Jung's view of the psyche (Jung, 1958). He distinguishes three psychological processes. The first, consciousness, contains the ego by which each person identifies himself. Then there is the personal unconscious which, like consciousness, is formed as each individual develops a personal history. However, the personal unconscious contains emotionally charged information repressed to sustain an ego-image in consciousness. Finally, the collective unconscious differs from the other two psychological processes because it is not formed from individual experiences. Instead, according to Jung, it is determined by the human species' evolutionary development and contains brain patterns for the most intense emotional responses which humans experience.

Jung's analysis of the psyche parallels the hero's journey as delineated by Campbell (1968). People live with their conscious egos, Campbell states, until a crisis occurs and acts as a "call" to begin the hero's journey. The "call" is any life-event or series of events which challenges assumptions people have about their ego-identities. The journey itself starts with explorations of the personal unconscious and its repressed emotions. Bringing these emotions to consciousness expands the base of ego-identity, enabling it to include more and more information which had been repressed. Once the hero consciously accepts formerly unconscious material, according to Jung and Campbell, he encounters the emotions which comprise the collective unconscious. At this deep unconscious level, he can deal with the fundamental issues of his existence and complete his journey by bringing the gifts of his new awareness to the world.

THE CONSCIOUSNESS/EGO CHALLENGED

Before the journey begins, it is necessary to understand the nature of the consciousness which Jung and Campbell state will eventually be transformed. The conscious or ego-identity is comprised of the many roles people play. Unless a person has entered the ranks of the "self-actualized," "individuated" or "enlightened," he uses information from his environment in a continuous loop of negative and positive feedback to solidify for himself who he is and who he is not. For instance, he plays the role of a good son and his family's approval affirms this. The death of his parents destroys a portion of that approval feedback loop, affecting his ego-identity and compelling him to redefine who he is. Redefinition, then, is one of the keys to transformation through grief and loss (Bowlby, 1980).

Grief, in this model, is the response of the ego loosened from an essential identity mooring and cast adrift in uncertainty. People grieve to the extent that their ego-identity is invested in the lost relationship. A portion of their grief reaction is their inability to really know who they are without this role-defining feedback. However, being willing to suspend their identity, that is being willing to endure the confusion of not knowing exactly who they are anymore, is the first step in redefinition. This confusion, however, often presents frightening psychological possibilities for the individual.

This was, for example, the experience of a widow who had been happily married for nearly 20 years. She was involved with her children's school, drove them to their lessons, and acted as a Cub Scout Leader. She considered herself a good wife and a good mother. Her husband had no complaints; she gave him support when things went wrong at work and was a delightful companion and a gracious hostess. She followed his lead in almost everything, even their friends were his work associates. Whenever a crisis arose, no matter how trivial, he was the one who decided the course of action for them to take.

When he became ill with inoperable cancer, she was almost paralyzed with fear. She only knew herself as someone who calmly and graciously did things to please others. She made decisions, of course, on what color draperies to buy and where in the yard to plant flowers, but she never challenged his decision-making authority. He liked her that way and his approval reinforced her identity. As he became weaker and needed her to manage their affairs, she no longer got his approval for being dependent. Instead, he expected her to make decisions and take care of everything, including him. He became angry at her uncertainties and hesitancy.

With this change in his priorities, one of her former approval-feedback loops had been broken and she could not function according to her previous identity. But how was she to function? His mixed messages had completely confused her. Her journey began when she answered the "call," forcing herself to meet the needs of the situation, no longer the docile wife, but not sure of what she would become.

THE PERSONAL UNCONSCIOUS/
IDENTITY CONFUSION

Part of the confusion connected with the suspension of identity comes from some of the alternative roles which emerge from the personal unconsciousness. Jung calls this repressed information the "shadow" of the ego (Jung, 1971). Shadow began to develop during the early years of childhood when family, peers, and society defined who the widow was in relation to the roles she played in their lives. She secretly knew she was often something other than what she was told she should be and the emotions surrounding this other part of herself were repressed into her shadow.

As part of the repression of these unwelcomed aspects of herself, various psychological mechanisms appeared. Called ego-defense mechanisms, they protected her from the frightening possibility that the shadow would emerge and threaten both her ego-image and her relationships with those who would disapprove of her shadow side.

As her husband became a hospice patient and then died, she lost the role of dependent helpmate. This left a gap in her self-image and her protective mechanisms lost some of their ability to defend her ego against its shadow. As a result, some secret, shadow qualities escaped from the personal unconscious and more of who she really was began to emerge. Because this kind of information came to her ego as unknown elements of the psyche, they resembled the unknown generally, and posed a threat to her survival. In answering the "call" and facing the challenge of a new situation, the widow displayed more courage than she had ever dreamed possible.

The independent part of her personality had been consciously denied in order to maintain her relationships with her family and then her husband, but it still existed in the unconscious parts of her psyche, emerging in dreams and fantasies which her consciousness had trouble understanding.

Early in her grieving process, the widow dreamed of an aggressive, competent businesswoman she knew. The woman in her dream insulted the widow and chased her through the rooms of a big, old house. The businesswoman was, according to Jung, the widow's shadow — her own capacity for being independent and competent which she had denied. In this model, her dream was suggesting to her that she was as assertive and competent as the businesswoman, while the chase meant she was still denying her capacity to assert herself. This capacity was literally chasing through her psyche, looking for a new definition of who she would become.

In Jung's view, the businesswoman in the widow's dream was not someone separate from her, but an aspect of herself which she had strong, emotional reasons for denying. More specifically, female assertiveness was not respected by her family, so the widow had projected her unacknowledged or "unowned" shadow onto the businesswoman who then symbolized the widow's *fear* of the responsibilities inherent in being independent and competent. At this point in her life, she not only didn't know who she was, but feared both what she might have to become and what her family's response might be to this change.

According to Jung, this shadow dream arose from the personal unconscious, the widow's unique history. Before the widow could redefine herself, this aspect of her shadow had to be experienced. In experiencing her shadow, not only must she intellectually acknowledge, "Well yes, I could really do everything I need in order to survive," but she must also incorporate that information into her life-style. In other words, she must experience the emotions around assertiveness which she had so neatly repressed during her childhood. Along with redefinition and suspension of the ego, experiencing formerly repressed emotions is seen as another vital part of the transformation process.

The fears awakened by emerging shadow material are too much for some people to handle and many mourners refuse to deal with them. For instance, a bereaved mother may persist in her role as her dead son's mother by communing regularly with his spirit through the efforts of a trance medium. Campbell (1968) refers to such denials as "refusing the call" to the journey of transformation. Jung (1971) describes the process as inflation or depression of the ego.

The inflated response occurs when someone takes a small revelation from the personal unconscious, thinks it is from the collective unconscious and calls it "Truth." Then, Jung says, he feels no need to deal with any other shadow information. The grieving mother who consulted the trance medium exemplified inflation when she went to bereavement group meetings and tried to convince others to make contact with their dead family members. She had the Truth and they should acknowledge it.

With ego depression, Jung says, an individual assumes his own shadow characterizes humans generally and therefore all is lost. The widow described above would have been in this category if she had taken her husband's death as an indication that she could not depend on anybody or anything, that she is merely a victim of some impersonal power. Then from her perceived victimization, she would have regarded this as characteristic of the human experience where people have no hope of happiness. This would be her Truth and, in this hypothetical scenario, those who love her would undoubtably try, but fail, to convince her that she is wrong.

Those with both ego inflation and depression maintain a kind of superiority because they believe only they have information beyond ego-consciousness itself. Due to their repression of the shadow's emotionally-charged content, they continue to play their former ego roles, augmented only by their brief glimpses into the personal unconscious. No ego redefinition occurs and they lose the opportunity for transformation.

Hospice caregivers encountering inflation or depression should recognize that the function of these responses is a defensive, protective one. Most people, Jung (1971) points out, will stay with these defensive devices until they acquire the courage to again suspend their ego-identities. A characteristic of these defensive responses is their intractability. Until people are ready to move, attempts to prod them into continuing the journey merely produce anger. Their augmented ego-identities seem so right to them that the prod is taken as a challenge to their Truth.

It is best to wait for clues that the time for change has come. For some people, it may take another crisis, another "call," before the process can resume and lead to transformation. The "call" can be detected through fantasies and dreams, such as the chase in the widow's dream which meant the process toward growth had been activated, but was stalled while she searched for a direction to take.

The painfulness of redefinition may begin for some bereaved during a month to six weeks crisis point following the death of a family member. At this time, the work of settling the departed's affairs usually has been accomplished and grief is intensified as day-to-day activities resume without the ego-defining relationship. At this point in the widow's grieving process, a hospice bereavement counselor helped her by encouraging honesty about her perceived needs and openness to clues which indicated the nature of the issues — shadow material — with which she was dealing. Using the chase dream and others, the counselor helped the widow understand some of her own resources for building a new life. She needed encouragement, almost permission, to integrate the emerging information from the personal unconscious into her conscious ego-identity. With that integration came part of the needed redefinition, allowing her to acknowledge she is more than just the former roles she had played.

As she encountered her shadow and was willing to recognize another part of herself, expanding her definition of who she is in the process, the widow began her journey through grief. This loosened the hold of both the certainties of the ego and its reliance on defense mechanisms of the personal unconscious. Once she had acknowledged another possible way of being, she tacitly gave permission for the emergence of even more of her repressions. This meant she would eventually come face-to-face with the transpersonal, existential issues of the collective unconscious, those issues which relate to the meaning of life.

THE COLLECTIVE UNCONSCIOUS/ DISCOVERING MEANING

Jung states that humans are psychologically linked together through the processes of the collective unconscious. These processes represent species-unique brain patterns for responding to existential questions — who we are, why we were born, and what will become of us. Our similar responses are recorded, Jung says, in the religions and mythologies of the world. The evolutionary process uniquely provided humans with brains which enable us to ask these questions and, in order to enhance psychological survival, Jung reasoned, other brain processes must be available to provide the answers. Otherwise, our brains, which allow us to reason from cause to effect, would have left us floundering in existential despair, psychologically paralyzed and unable to provide for our biological survival.

Just as the personal unconscious is presented to consciousness as projections of the shadow, the collective unconscious is revealed through symbols of the archetypes (Jung, 1971). Archetype is Jung's term for the emotional responses which accompany the human quest for the meaning of life. By understanding the significance of archetypal symbols, we find answers to the existential questions. Archetypal symbols appear in dreams and fantasies, just as the shadow representations do, and may well have done so since the beginning of humankind. Many of the symbols which express the truths of the world's religions and fill the dreams of modern humans have been preserved for at least 60,000 years in emotionally charged myths, rituals, and images of our ancient ancestors. Such an ancient symbol still survives in the use of flowers for human burials.

The report of a profoundly "religious" dream by a bereaved person should alert a counselor to the possibility of an archetypal dream. Another characteristic of archetypal dreams is the preponderance of unknown people and places, although known elements may also appear in more secondary roles. The grieving widow, for instance, in telling of a "religious" dream she had, was signalling that she was ready to deal with archetypal issues.

Just as the widow's perception of herself as a docile homebody was challenged by the realities of her husband's death, so were her relationships to the world and to her own life. She had grown up assuming that if she just did what she was told she would be loved and wouldn't be alone or rejected. This gave her some control over what she most feared. Then her husband's death occurred and she was unprepared for the destruction of that myth. She could no longer behave in the way that had previously given her a sense of control. The answers to her existential questions no longer worked, in part because she had found them in her family and husband and not in herself. She needed new answers and to find them she had to complete the first phase of her journey (Campbell, 1968) and then continue on.

Previously, in her journey, she had only dealt with the defense mechanisms and repressed shadow which had protected her ego from disturbing archetypal issues. The transformations of some shadow brought about changes in the roles she assumed but, with encountering the archetypes, she would move beyond roles to the very essence of being human. At this point, defense mechanisms are no longer needed because there are no roles here. There are only humans who relate to the world and to other humans at the most elementary level of their existence. Here the widow would have to acknowledge her connection to that level of being which transcends all cultures and the roles they impose on us.

Continuing her journey, the widow encountered the two major archetypes involved in transformation. These represent the polarities of human experience and are depicted through masculine and feminine symbols; hence they are named the masculine and feminine archetypes. Together these archetypes symbolize the elemental relationships of human beings and answer the questions, "Am I, as a human being, unique in the universe? Or am I, as a human being, part of nature which merely comes into existence and then dies?" A connection to the world's religions is obvious because they too strive to answer these same questions, questions raised through the influence of the archetypes.

THE FEMININE ARCHETYPE/ DISCOVERING LINKS TO NATURE

In mythological terms, encountering the feminine archetype at this phase of the journey is described as meeting the goddess and the temptress (Campbell, 1968). The feminine archetypal processes are those which the hero experiences as a necessary biological connection to nature, a connection which generates contradictory emotions. There is awe and wonder at the mystery and miracle of birth and nurture, especially at the breast. These emotions are mingled with fear as the cycles of life impersonally proceed through the realm of death.

This connection to the natural world means that we humans are born through no effort of our own, are nourished and then die by the whims of nature—or as the Hindus say, life is merely a game played by Brahman, the universal creator. Underlying our fear of death is the need to control our destinies so we are not as helpless as, for instance, the antelope grazing as a lion approaches. Because of our brains, we want more answers and more control than the brain of the antelope demands. Humans ultimately have little control over the process of life and, like the antelope, no power to avert death. Nature decides this through the limits set on the assaults safely endured by the human body.

When the widow grieved, she grieved for the loss of her ego-identifying relationship and the loss of the fiction that she could control her life. Like her, we are not prepared in our culture for this eternal process of life and death. Western religious traditions have been built on the premise that, if we did what was prescribed, we would not die. We would not suffer the most devastating loss, the death of our personal egos or souls.

Dream images which symbolize the feminine have a threefold nature, corresponding to the Triple Goddess of the ancient world. A crone with empty breasts and womb appeared in the widow's dreams shortly after her husband's death. According to Jung, it symbolized the death of her old ego-identity as it faded away. Later, she had a series of dreams with young women or virgins (in the ancient meaning, that of a woman who was not yet a mother) offering to help her out of various difficulties. At this time, the widow had made plans to use some of her husband's insurance money in order to take a secretarial course. A new life was taking shape, symbolized by the womb of young women ready to start the process of bringing forth.

Coupled with dreams of young women were other dreams of a young child or infant. At first the child was buried under dirt or piles of things and the widow would see herself frantically trying to free the child. Eventually, her child, her new conscious identity, was brought forth and nurtured. In some dreams, this was literally presented as suckling, but in others she was given gifts which allowed her to solve some problems and grow in confidence. In her life, she was also finding ways to solve problems—those of a single parent, a working mother and an unmarried woman. In her dreams, the emotionally laden information about the changes in her life were presented to her through the symbols of the feminine archetype.

In the process of life and death which is represented by the Triple Goddess, the virgin is transformed into the nourishing mother who suckles and protects the infant, her new ego-identity. In the widow's dreams, the nourishing mother is none other than that part of herself which can meet her own needs and allow her to continue growing. But if transformation is to reach its greatest heights, then the nourishing mother will inevitably be transformed into the death crone as the widow experiences the inappropriateness of even her new ego-identity. She will die again and again to any incomplete definition of who she is as the cycle of the ego's life, death, and rebirth mirrors the cycle of nature, eternally perpetuating itself.

Bereaved persons often report death symbols in their dreams. For instance, Edgar Jackson reported the dream of a woman whose husband had died. She dreamed that she had pulled him apart from limb to limb (a death image), trying to fit him into a suitcase so that she could move to a new home. By the woman's own analysis of the dream, she recognized that she had to give up her husband's personal things and move without them into her new home in order to make a fresh start (Jackson, 1977).

The death aspect of the feminine must be experientially integrated, just as shadow material was owned. The widow did this by experiencing her connection to the unending cycle of the natural world—the seasons, the sun and moon, all of which are born and die along with living things. Again, Jung would say, it is necessary for the widow to experience the emotions from her unconscious, only this time the emotions are generated from unresolved issues around the archetypal processes.

Many people intellectually acknowledge their biological connection to nature, but will not allow themselves to experience the existential angst of death and dying. Angst is born from that sickening realization that we, too, ultimately have no control over our lives. Our loved ones die, and we will die, all according to nature's plan. Accepting the feminine means accepting this part of our reality, our biological bond to the earth, and saying, "That's OK; I'll go on anyway."

Some people will use religious concepts and terminology to describe this realization. Others will look more directly at their connections to nature and other life forms. Whatever the framework used to describe the response, it transforms.

THE MASCULINE ARCHETYPE/
DISCOVERING LINKS TO OTHERS

But the journey isn't over. Next, Campbell points out, the hero meets the masculine archetype and "atones with the father" (Campbell, 1968). Again looking to the ancient world, the masculine appears through symbols of the gods. These gods were once tribal or nature gods who protected ancient clans and guided the paleolithic hunters, providing the focus around which life in human society was bound together in mutual support. In unique and powerful ways, they represent that special human bonding which values the individual, but also allows him to sacrifice himself to sustain the group.

The masculine archetype is the psychological process which embodies emotions generated by the realization that each person is unique, that humans as a species are unique and somehow experience themselves as more than just their biology. Humans, after all, don't merely adapt to nature but adapt nature to themselves, appearing almost like the gods. Our paleolithic ancestors learned to cultivate and regulate the production of grain supplies and to hunt with traps, tracking, and weapons which were all devised by them. They knew that they had power in the natural world, but not just as individuals. Since prehistory human power has been manifested through unique bonds formed with other humans, enabling them to cooperatively perform life-sustaining activities. Such purposes and understanding of uniqueness continues to link humans to each other in ways different from the bonds formed by any other member of the animal kingdom, even other mammals.

In the widow's dreams, the unknown male figures representing the masculine archetype often appeared. Initially, these men chased, eluded or threatened her, as she devoted herself almost exclusively to her studies and her family. Once her husband was gone, she discovered that she could no longer be part of the couples scene and this upset her. She had not previously realized their friends were really his friends, but became painfully aware of this through their indifference once the funeral was over. She withdrew into her own world and, in an almost complete about-face, decided she needed no one; she could carry on alone. Eventually, she met some interesting women and then some men. She was no longer dependent on them for support and so she saw them in new ways. For the first time in her life, she accepted their caring and reached out in true friendship, just as an unknown man in one of her dreams reached out and offered her a glass of wine.

THE APOTHEOSIS OF THE HERO/ PSYCHOLOGICAL INTEGRATION

Together, the masculine and feminine archetypes represent the last monumental task of redefinition required for transformation of the hero—to experience simultaneously both horns of the human paradox. This involves emotionally validating both the impersonal processes of nature which link us to other life forms and the personal processes of the human community by expressing uniquely human characteristics—reasoning, inventiveness, and compassion. In other words, powerful and vulnerable at the same time, the widow experienced herself as part of nature, and yet somehow understood that she transcends it.

In the transpersonal model, the widow's journey at this point had reached a stage of integration (Campbell, 1968). Although sensing a powerful transformation in her life, she became increasingly aware that there were still many things for her to learn about herself. By "meeting" other "calls," embarking on several other journeys into her unconscious, she would become increasingly transformed into ever new levels of self-awareness. Her dreams would eventually begin to present symbols of wholeness, such as mandalas (usually geometric forms with perfect symmetry), integrated masculine and feminine images or images which represent the union of opposites.

The stage would be set for a hero's (in her case a heroine's) apotheosis with an awareness of her oneness with nature enhanced by her compassion for the strength and vulnerability of humans. The task of an ideal lifetime, this stage is characterized by the "return" and should the widow eventually reach it, she would bring gifts to the world, gifts which all may not understand (Campbell, 1968). She would gradually abandon any vestiges of role-playing and no longer need feedback from others in order to define herself. Some would become uncomfortable with her because they are only capable of relating to themselves and others through their various roles. She would accept them as human beings and they may not understand what that means.

Even though the process of transformation in this model has been described here as linear, in actuality it is circular. Bereaved persons may start the journey several times and get stuck, having to begin the process again at a later date. Even though Jung states that the shadow must first be experienced before the hero can start to deal with the collective unconscious, he does not mean the hero must completely resolve shadow issues before he can start dealing with archetypes. The circular, spiraling process of transformation continuously carries the psyche through both personal and collective unconscious issues.

Dreams also reflect this circularity with dreams one night being personal, the next night being archetypal and maybe the next night mixed personal and archetypal. The understanding and awareness which comes from each kind of dream enhances the processes presented by the other.

At each time the widow was challenged to redefine who she is, the opportunity for transformation was reawakened. With each redefinition, she acknowledged more and more shadow while experiencing, with increasing clarity, the existential realities of the archetypes.

This means that, to the extent she accepts or owns her shadow, she is more open to material from the archetypes. To the extent that she connects with the natural cycles of the feminine, she is more aware of her masculine humanness. To the extent that she feels bonded in compassion to the uniqueness and vulnerability of her fellow humans, she experiences both her connection and theirs to the natural world. And, finally, to the extent that she connects with nature and her fellow humans, she can accept her shadow and love herself, even though she knows she isn't perfect.

Many who have suffered great losses and then experienced transformation describe experiences similar to those of encountering the

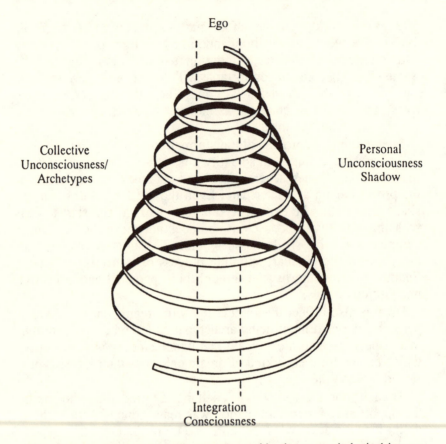

Figure 1. Jungian Components of the Psyche

Consciousness develops away from mere ego identity as psychological integration occurs. As it moves away from ego identity, it absorbs increasingly more of both kinds of unconscious repressions, expanding individual awareness and minimizing rol playing.

shadow and archetypes. "Many widows with whom I have spoken have described their period of grief as a time of intensified growth and understanding, even though it was also a period of intensified pain and confusion" (Moody, 1977; 18). Their testimony points to the value of exploring further the possibilities of using Jung's and Campbell's model. With an understanding of both these theories and the corresponding psychodynamics of the grieving process, both caregivers and their patients/families may be able to expand their ability to turn grief into personal transformation, thereby turning the mourner into the hero.

REFERENCES

Bowlby, J. (1980) *Loss: Sadness and Depression* (Vol III) New York: Basic Books.

Campbell, J. (1968) *The Hero with a Thousand Faces* (2nd Ed.) Princeton, NJ: Princeton University Press.

Campbell, J. (Ed.) (1971) *The Portable Jung* New York: Viking.

de Laszlo, V.S. (Ed.) (1958) *Psyche and Symbol: A Selection from the Writings of C. G. Jung* New York: Doubleday Anchor.

Jackson, Edgar. (1957) *Understanding Grief* New York: Abingdon Press.

Moody, J.M. (1977) "Dreaming and Bereavement" *Pastoral Psychology* 26(1) (pp. 12-21.)

Bereavement Groups
in the Hospice Program

Joan S. Buell
Jeanne Bevis

SUMMARY. This article reviews the nature of the therapeutic activity in bereavement groups — the rationale behind offering them in a hospice program for the general public — and then looks specifically at bereavement programs offered at Hospice House in Portland, Oregon. It covers eligibility, attendance, issues, methods used to consolidate the groups, blending of new members, and specifies the types of groups involved. Further, it explores the formation of a city-wide bereavement network, formed to provide mutual support for facilitators and counselors to exchange ideas, shape continuing education, encourage cross-referral and avoid duplication.

The founding principle behind the support group is that human beings who have experienced a given condition can truly empathize and "know" what another individual is going through when they

Joan S. Buell, MA, is Executive Director of the Hospice House in Portland, OR, a freestanding hospice which opened in September, 1987. She has served as a counselor there and was formerly Director of Volunteers for a homecare hospice team. She worked for five months as a volunteer nursing assistant at St. Christopher's in London and directly observed the bereavement program of Dr. Colin Murray Parkes. She has published in the field of child development and hospice care. Jeanne Bevis, MSW, RCSW, is a counselor with the Arigo counseling team at Hospice House. She also works part-time for Kaiser Permanente in the Cancer Counseling Center. Ms. Bevis has a long history of professional experience in the mental health field and maintains a psychotherapeutic private practice, seeing individuals, couples, and families for a variety of mental health needs. Address correspondence to the authors at Hospice House, 6171 SW Capitol Highway, Portland, OR.

are in that condition. And it is the sense of empathy and shared experience that participants search for as an assuaging element in a group (Kirschling & Akers, 1986). Some eventual alleviation of pain occurs as people find themselves less isolated and can put their own pain in a larger context, even in the case of bereaved families who choose to participate in a group with other families (Elde, 1986).

The group, in the context of a hospice program's bereavement follow-up, can be viewed as a logical extension of the notes, telephone calls, social gatherings and home visits already provided. The purpose of this paper is to review briefly the function and therapeutic activity of a bereavement group, to describe the practice of offering groups in a hospice program, and finally to encourage the formation of community-wide bereavement counselors' networks.

THE NATURE
OF THE THERAPEUTIC ACTIVITY
OF A BEREAVEMENT GROUP

Bereavement groups have particular qualities. The individuals are not coping with an identifiable illness such as alcoholism or multiple sclerosis but with a condition that to some feels, at worst, like an illness and, in any case, like a pervading "craziness," full of overwhelming and unmanageable feelings. They have been thrust into role changes and financial obligations. Besides the new activities required of them, it is what is not happening that is a major part of the problem.

As bereaved individuals they are searching for affirmation, validation and often education. They want to know more about what is happening to them and to learn how to survive it. There are tantalizing dichotomies for many individuals. They expect to find a similarity of experience among the group members, and at the same time want to hear that their experience is unique. They search for relief from pain even as they put themselves in a position of reliving painful experiences and being near the pain of others. At times, a person finding someone who has had an experience very close to their own sees that the similarity only serves to accentuate what is unique about each one. For example, the loss of a child for one couple may have precipitated a divorce, whereas for another it may have drawn the pair closer. One woman, during the early stages of her husband's Alzheimer's disease, may have found her friends increasingly helpful and attentive. For another it may have been a time of progressive isolation which pushed her into substance abuse.

There are common feelings and experiences identified by various members of a group, that when spoken out loud, allow an individual to muse, "Oh, that's right, that's how I feel." This identification of thoughts and feelings, and subsequent normalization, provides relief and allows the person to say "Oh, I'm ok, I'm not going crazy." Feelings of "I'm not normal" or "I am, or might be going, crazy" are common among individuals facing extreme stress. This reassurance that one is alright is likely to be one of the significant contributions a group has to offer, for "If these thoughts and feelings are normal, and others can survive and heal, then so can I."

The actual therapeutic activity in a group bears some similarity to paradoxical intervention. Rather than urging the individual to change, the facilitator and members of the group are actually affirming the individual's need to continue to feel the same way for the time being. To create the impression that they shouldn't be feeling as they do right now might be doing them a disservice. The griever is best served who receives from others permission and encouragement to explore, delineate, and describe the feelings that are emerging at the moment. Through this exploration, the individual further has the opportunity both to express feelings and to find ways of managing them to meet life demands. Perhaps for this reason, those professionals in the community who assume that change is desirable and desired often find it difficult to allow the grieving person sufficient time to do the work required.

The ability of the group to allow time for grieving may be another of its major strengths. Long after a grieving person has tired family and friends with their constant ruminations, a group can stay with that person. Healing can require a witness to the pain and grief. Others going through the experience can provide inexhaustible, attentive witness and support.

HOSPICE AS A SITE FOR BEREAVEMENT GROUPS

Churches (Sklar & Huneke, 1987), senior centers and hospitals are frequently sites for bereavement groups, with each one bringing a particular orientation of their own. Death is a part of everyday life for hospices. Neither hurrying nor prolonging a process is the rule. It is a logical place for a bereavement group that extends beyond the families and friends of those who have died in the hospice program. Counselors who have experience with the issues of loss are already present. The community begins to call on the hospice program because it knows that hospice care has something to do with death. Frequently, in a small city, the hospice program is one of the few places where intricate knowledge of grief and all its ramifications exists at the professional level. Social workers or mental health professionals in the community may also offer their services through the hospice on a part-time basis. They may do this, after a careful selection process, as volunteers or for nominal payment. This may serve for the professional, too, as a way of confirming their affinity with the philosophy of serving the community, and broadening their own skills. They can serve as individual counselors or as group facilitators. At regular meetings with hospice staff, they can provide mutual support and supervision.

Hospice House began in 1980, operating out of one small room in an old Portland, Oregon home. Helping families to care for the dying, using volunteers, was the first service offered. Early on, Hospice House recognized the need for counseling services and developed a small counseling program known as Arigo (Arigo means "help" in Greek). The need for bereavement group services also became immediately apparent, and Hospice House subsequently began offering these groups. As the need for services grew, Hospice House grew as well, building the first freestanding, 15-bed, inpatient hospice facility in Oregon. Expanded services further required new guidelines for eligibility, screening, enrollment and attendance, based on community needs and activities at Hospice House.

The city of Portland already claimed three (now six) hospice home-care teams based in hospitals and a home health agency. In the last seven years Hospice House and these teams have trained their volunteers together, held monthly network exchange meetings and have participated along with other hospices from across Oregon in the writing of standards for hospice care in the state.

Each is a separate corporate entity, all accredited by the Oregon Hospice Association according to the above mentioned standards, which are recognized by the state and Blue Cross. Hospice House is also licensed by the state as a freestanding hospice facility under new rules written by the Oregon State Health Division in 1987.

Realizing there was a need in the community for open bereavement services and that Hospice House could provide these through partially-donated professional time, the Arigo program began seeing individual clients and offering groups in 1982, long before the freestanding building was a reality. The facilitators gathered, established policies and developed a sense of cooperation and mutual supervision.

Funding came first from donations to cover minimal costs. Later Hospice House received a grant to fund the counseling program. This grant continues to be used for individuals seeking group or individual counseling who are completely unable to pay. For those able to afford some level of payment, sliding fees were established by comparison with accepted citywide counseling pay scales.

The decision to provide facilitators rather than to use a participant-run format sprang from several considerations. Observation showed that many participant-run groups dissolved when the needs of the prime movers had been met. The intricacy of interaction required a skilled person, to avoid monopolization, to be alert to complications that might require referral, to bring clear information, and to provide continuity. The pairing of facilitators gives each of them back-up, mutual supervision and also a lessening of the burden to provide continuity for every meeting.

Eligibility

The chief criterion for participation in the group is having experienced a loss through death. The time elapsed since the death, it appears, is not particularly relevant, with one possible exception. The individual who is still in a state of shock, and joins the group in the very first weeks after the death, may not be able to find what is needed. This person, hearing the emotionally painful stories of other group members may feel completely overwhelmed and leave the group. If the person needs to talk steadily and without interruption, it is difficult to meet that need and at the same time allow all members of the group a chance to be heard. And yet, if they want to sit silent and absorb the sounds of those around them, it may be that hearing the voices of other survivors is actually one path to confirming the reality.

Neither does there seem to be a maximum limit on the time since the death. One family member came to the Survivors of Suicide group 25 years after the suicide of her husband. She was able to resolve her deeply-felt guilt and anger in group after all those years.

Because the bereaved person has decided to come into a social situation out of a condition of comparative isolation, the action itself is significant. It puts the person in a place where they can justifiably talk about, be angry at, or weep for, a person who isn't there. In the group they can find confirmation that those activities are worth doing, and that they are healthy.

Screening and Enrollment

A person calls and states that they wish to join the group. Often during that first conversation the bereaved person gleans information about the program and also gives some information about himself/herself. These conversations are not handled by the receptionist at the Hospice House because so often they become quite long and occasionally emotional. The receptionist connects the call with a staff designee (rotating) who completes an initial referral form. The information then goes to one of the two facilitators of the appropriate group. A facilitator calls each applicant and determines if that person is appropriate for the group. Criteria for appropriateness would include the following:

1. An expressed desire to be with others in a group experience.
2. No evidence of a psychotic disorder; if this becomes difficult to determine, a brief mental health history is taken, and inquiries are made into previous mental health treatment.
3. No evidence of drug or alcohol addiction. If questionable, appropriate history is taken and inquiries are made.

4. Some ability to express relevant thoughts and feelings about the death. Individuals are not required to be highly verbal, but group experience does require some sharing eventually by all members.

If there is some doubt, the facilitator may request a personal interview. Or, if the group is full, and several people are waiting to join it already, the individual may be offered a session alone with the facilitator so that they will not have to forego support when they have asked for it. Since the bereaved person has mustered the energy and courage it takes to make the initial call it is advisable not to put them off, if possible. The facilitator, in some cases, may recommend referral for therapy and not accept the person into the group until their therapist recommends that it will be helpful.

Attendance

For the first four sessions, the individual is asked to attend sequentially, for two reasons. The first session, for many people, proves extremely painful because issues are often being voiced for the first time. The vividness of the loss returns. It is as though the death had happened yesterday. The pain is great enough to make the person feel they don't want to submit themselves to it again. Secondly, bonds and the sense of community with other members of the group have not had a chance to develop until several sessions have been completed, so there is nothing to counteract that initial pain.

Asking a person to come four times consecutively upon entering the group has several positive effects. The person seriously considers how strongly he/she feels about making this step of joining the group. They are less likely to treat it as a drop-in, casual glimpse. The facilitator discusses with the applicant the possibility that the first few sessions will be painful and that the pain may seem to outweigh the therapeutic value at first. Prepared in this way, the new group member can weather the strangeness and freshening of the pain, enduring until the period when the new bonds they form with other group members become enriching and palliative in themselves.

From that time on, the agreements are as follows:

- Call the facilitator if you plan to be absent.
- Let the group know ahead of time if you plan to stop coming for good, so they can say goodbye.
- Let the group know if small subgroups are getting together for socializing between group meetings.

Further along in a person's participation, certain group members have reported that, at particularly bad times, they have stayed away from the group temporarily. One way the group has addressed this phenomenon, recognizing that it has happened to more than one member, is agreeing they will at least call another member of the group when the desire to isolate themselves occurs.

Many members of groups form individual alliances. Frequently, group members request phone numbers of other group members in order to keep in contact and reach out when needed between sessions. These alliances are extremely helpful to both isolated individuals who don't have support systems, as well as to individuals who have family and friends, but who just need to talk to someone not connected with their network.

Whether a bereaved person chooses group or individual counseling will probably depend on personality factors as much as anything else. Those who find group activity attractive as such would be more likely to gravitate to the bereavement group. The more private person would find the validation and sharing easier to accept in a one-to-one situation.

Consolidating the Group

A group which has difficulty gaining cohesiveness can be stopped and restarted only when the firm number of attendees for the new group has risen to ten or so. During the first few sessions under this new form, the facilitators slightly increase the structure at the start of each session by focusing on a particular issue, using handouts to stimulate discussion and give information. Important group personal bonds begin to form. The group is returned to its preferred non-agenda format but does not go back to its non-cohesive character.

Less threatening for some than a "group," with its connotations of self-revelation and confrontation, is the idea of calling a group a "class." There are continuing reports that the "class," starting out with a relatively didactic format, often converts itself into a support group and becomes, in spite of the original intent, an ongoing entity. Nothing is lost. Some social interactions grow out of what has been generated in the initial meetings, while those who wish to stop can do so.

THE NEWLY BEREAVED
ENTERING AN OPEN-ENDED GROUP

Facilitators and group members search for comfortable and responsible ways to integrate the newly bereaved into what may have become a tightly knit group. If this is not done well, the new arrivals can experience a sense of isolation that they little need. They may also be surprised at the intensity of feelings in people who have had losses some years before. These realizations may serve as confirmation that there is indeed work to be done and that the present is a good time to do it.

The facilitator needs to be aware, however, that it can also serve to scare newcomers, leaving them with the feeling that "If it goes on this long, how can I survive?" plunging them into more hopelessness about their loss. If this is discussed openly in group, the old-timers often respond "You should have seen me a year ago." They can also share unique and creative secrets they have used for healing themselves, offering support that is different from that provided by the newly-bereaved because it includes the knowledge of the waves of pain. "Old-timers" who are beginning to rebuild their lives present a clear picture to the newly-bereaved that it is possible to fully participate in life again.

Methods that have proved successful for integrating newcomers include bringing into the group only one — or at the most two — new people at a time. This allows the older group members time to attend to the new member(s), as well as to continue the group's well-established patterns. Another helpful method is structuring the introductions so that each old member shares with the new member their reasons for being in the group and what the group has meant to them. It also seems extremely important that the new members share with the group at least something about their reasons for coming (i.e., who they've lost and how). Even reluctant new members feel a sense of bonding if it is expected that they share some minimal information. The group then has an opportunity to empathize with them and group process begins.

TYPES OF GROUPS OFFERED
AT HOSPICE HOUSE

A weekly evening bereavement group has been in continuous existence for four years now. Members of this group have had varied losses and are at varied distances in time from those losses. Some members attend specific-loss groups such as Compassionate Friends, or a church group, as well as attending this one. The weekly meeting has been a factor for some in making that decision since they need something more frequent than a monthly meeting.

The Survivors of Loss through Suicide (SOS) group meets twice monthly, also in the evenings. While this type of loss seems less closely related to hospice care, the need in the community-at-large was acute. The group has become a solid part of the Arigo program. There were several suicide prevention services in the area, but nothing for those who have been forced into the complicated grief caused by a completed suicide and the societal limbo that can follow.

Hospice House has most recently started a group for family and friends of those who are in the throws of life-threatening illness in its later stages. There are several cancer support groups in the area and a hospice is not necessarily an appropriate place for a group of individuals who are coping with the early stages of disease. But the growing intensity of anticipatory grief when the person is closer to dying has prompted many to call and ask for a group for persons at the later stage. Again, this group is open to the significant others of patients in the inpatient facility as well as to the larger community.

Hospice House's bereavement follow-up program for patients' families is given without charge. This includes a bereavement assessment done before the patients' death and immediately after, followed by telephone calls, notes, occasional home visits and the remembrance gatherings held twice yearly. The groups are offered with a small charge and on a sliding scale. Those for whom it is not a hardship pay a maximum of $10 per session. Others are assessed on a sliding fee scale.

BEREAVEMENT NETWORK

It is worthwhile considering the role of the hospice bereavement counseling program in the larger life of the community. Hospital social service programs and cancer rehabilitation programs, churches, public school counseling programs, funeral homes that have engaged a social worker or pastoral counselor to work with survivors, chaplaincy programs in hospitals — all these may be functioning in the community as resources for the bereaved. They may welcome participation by the hospice counselors and the formation of a bereavement counselors' network. Communication by mailings and meetings can save much time and duplication of services. Whoever takes the initiative, it is worth the effort.

Hospice House sponsored two counselors colloquia in 1982 and 1983. Subsequently, impetus came from other quarters, and in 1986 a small group brought together individuals from all areas where bereavement counseling was occurring.

The Bereavement Network meets quarterly, sharing information, previewing new materials and discussing particular counseling issues. Twice a year, network members also update and distribute a manual of the various resources available in Portland, Oregon and Vancouver, Washington for bereaved persons. This resource manual is available to nonmembers at cost. The meetings and the manual have provided good means for cross-referral, avoidance of duplication and an increased availability of services to the public.

Facilitating groups and being with people who are grieving can be emotionally exhausting work. Belonging to a bereavement network can provide support, nourishment and a sense of camaraderie that can help to sustain members during the weeks between meetings. Individuals and agencies rotate in carrying the administrative tasks, and there is an $8 annual fee for membership.

CONCLUSION

Bereavement groups have distinctive characteristics and by their nature can prove both enriching and draining for participants and facilitators. Hospice programs can reintegrate their hospice families into the larger community by merging hospice survivors with those who have had losses of these kinds in other places. And finally, above all, the returning joy seen in those who are beginning to reorganize and reinvest their affections is warming and reaffirming for all concerned.

An interaction between the hospice programs themselves, and between hospices and other agencies proves beneficial in many ways. These include the opportunity to teach, to serve the community and to enrich each other.

REFERENCES

Elde, C. (1986). The use of multiple group therapy in support groups for grieving families. *The American Journal of Hospice Care, 3*(6), 27-30.

Kirschling, J.M. & Akers, S. (1986). Group experience for the recently widowed. *The American Journal of Hospice Care, 3*(5), 24-27.

Parkes, C.M. (1981). Evaluation of a bereavement service. *Journal of Preventative Psychiatry, 1*(2), 179-187.

Sklar, F. & Huneke, K.D. (1987-1988). Bereavement: Ministerial attitudes and the future of church sponsored bereavement support groups. *Omega, 18*(2), 89-102.

Vachon, J.L.S., Lyall, W.A.L., Rogers, J., Freeman-Letofsky, K., & Freeman, S.J.J. (1980). A controlled study of self-help intervention for widows. *American Journal of Psychiatry, 137*, 1380-1384.

Vachon, M.L.S., Rogers, J., Lyall, W., Lancee, W.J., Sheldon, A.R., & Freeman, S.J.J. (1982). Predictors and correlates of adaptation to conjugal bereavement. *American Journal of Psychiatry, 139*, 998-1002.

The Volunteer in Bereavement Work: Tracking the Grief Process

Anne Compton

SUMMARY. A Hospice volunteer looks at common obstacles and challenges in the grief process for persons who have experienced the death of a loved one. Opportunities to give emotional support and appropriate information are offered to facilitate the volunteer's efforts in tracking the bereaved along the continuum of grief.

MY BACKGROUND IN HOSPICE

Almost ten years ago, I joined Boulder County Hospice in Boulder, Colorado as a volunteer. For over three years, I worked with terminally ill patients in their homes. I fed, bathed, and dressed people who had lost the power to do these simple things for themselves. In addition, we discussed their illness and its effects upon them and their loved ones. Strong bonds were forged between me, the patients, and their families in our struggle to preserve their relationships and the richness of their daily lives as we confronted the patients' pain, physical deterioration and, finally, death. To the dying all the valuable interactions they recall with their loved ones are precious memories – a bulwark of personal monuments attesting to love's power in the face of death.

Because of changes in my personal life in 1981, I turned my attention to the emotional impact of change and loss. I wondered how others met these challenges. In 1983 I left homecare with the dying and joined Hospice's bereavement team.

Anne Compton has been a volunteer with Boulder County Hospice since 1979. She has lectured extensively on bereavement to community groups. Also, she has helped in the training of public speakers and breavement workers.

Personal Expectations and Apprehensions

My expectation as a bereavement volunteer was that I would be able to facilitate the bereaved's expression of grief through active listening. I assumed that my presence alone would bring them some small measure of comfort. However, the devastation of personality that overwhelming grief brings was surprising to me. The death of a spouse or a child most often provokes this dramatic response. Since few people have knowledge of the grief process, the bereaved is usually ignored after the first few weeks. People often feel awkward or at a loss for words in confronting the grief of a friend or neighbor. I worried that I would not know what to say. I found out how important it is for each of us to at least acknowledge the loss by speaking a few words of condolence to the bereaved. Because grief is invisible, it is easy for the public to avoid any mention of it. Suffering arouses strong emotions in the people who witness it. Strong emotions are seldom expressed in a social context.

Before I began my work in bereavement, I worried that strong dependencies might result from sharing the intense feelings surrounding death and loss. Also, I wondered if my presence would be intrusive so soon after a family crisis. Traditionally, families close ranks and admit only close friends after a death (Bowlby, 1980).

Training and Assessment

Initially, my training in grief-work took place in bimonthly meetings of volunteers where our concerns were addressed by the supervisor. In addition, a chaplain and a social worker were present the first two years I was on the team. A psychiatrist also attended many of those meetings. Presently, a separate training in grief-work takes place for those interested in bereavement under the supervision of a social worker. The monthly meetings are attended by a psychologist who addresses any clinical issues.

Our meetings generally cover three areas: (a) our own personal obstacles in confronting the bereaved; (b) the special concerns of a particular person in grief; and (c) education on various aspects of grief.

Initial contacts with the bereaved are made by phone and most of the people I contact are flattered that Hospice still cares about them after the patient's death. In our program the volunteer usually tries to schedule a visit during the first or second phone conversation. An assessment of the degree of suffering and the effectiveness of the bereaved's coping skills help to determine to what extent the griever will need our support services. A home visit is the most effective way to assess the condition and lifestyle of the bereaved. Each volunteer has a checklist to determine the welfare of the bereaved.

Questions on this checklist concern changes in appetite, sleep habits, and weight. What drugs are used and how much alcohol is consumed also effect the bereaved's overall potential for adjustment. Furthermore, the volunteer needs to know about additional emotional burdens or physical problems that may complicate the grief process. Other questions determine the strength and durability of the support system. Usually, friends, family members, neighbors or clergy are part of the bereaved's community of support. Naturally, the volunteer's responsibility increases when the support system is weak or nonexistent, although the character and temperament of the bereaved are very significant in determining how well the challenges of grief will be met. It is important to encourage the bereaved to stay in contact with those people who encourage and support them. Many bereaved people worry excessively about imposing their sadness on others.

SIGNS AND SYMPTOMS OF GRIEF

The constancy of concern shown by the volunteer helps to stabilize the bereaved as they slowly make their way through the minefield of grief. Obstacles which may confront grievers include nightmares about the deceased, anxiety or panic attacks, feelings of unreality, an inability to concentrate or carry on the daily routine, and fatigue. The even more disturbing aspects of grief often involve parasensory experiences such as visions of the deceased, smelling an aroma from the past, or hearing the voice of the deceased. It is important that the volunteer ask about these experiences as the bereaved may not mention them for fear the volunteer may question their sanity.

One man said that his deceased wife was giving him advice about housework. He said he was greatly comforted by her voice, but he feared for his sanity. I assured him that many people in grief reported such incidents and that none had been insane (Parkes, 1972). On the contrary, this kind of event can be profoundly healing, making the loss itself easier to bear.

Violent or grisly circumstances surrounding a death exacerbate the difficulties facing the bereaved. One friend of mine, whose father committed suicide, remembers her shock at finding his glasses, blood-stained on the floor, where they had fallen after he had shot himself. This image intruded often on her thoughts, disturbing her for many months following his death. Symbols of tragedy haunt many bereaved people whose loved ones have died suddenly or in tragic circumstances. To share the pain of these upsetting memories is the job that volunteers do so well.

BEREAVEMENT TEAM GUIDELINES

A call approximately every four weeks and a visit at least twice a year is the average attention given to the bereaved by our team. Some get more, others less; however, if I feel any alarm on contacting a bereaved person, I consult my supervisor. Although it is hardly unusual for the bereaved to have occasional thoughts of suicide, I immediately report any intention or plan that is self-destructive. Alcohol problems or unforeseen crises (usually personal, financial or job-related) can put a staggering emotional burden on the already-exhausted person in grief. Crises require immediate attention. Any stressful change in addition to the death can trigger deep anxiety or panic. The response from the volunteer should be prompt, personal, and reassuring. All of the bereaved people I contact have my home phone number and I always ask them to call if they feel unduly distressed. This is the only way to ensure that emergencies will be addressed. In the last four years I have received fewer than six crisis calls. I also let the bereaved know they have access to professional therapists in emergencies as our Hospice has free crisis consultation services. The bereaved are also eligible for our monthly support groups.

Bereaved people need to be encouraged to grieve actively. To be sad or to cry in front of someone else is difficult for many adults.

Questions pertaining to the bereaved's welfare reassures them that you are sincerely interested and want to hear their story. If there is emotional conflict, the bereaved may become vague, evasive or hostile. I find that if I intervene and ask for clarification of something just said, the bereaved person has time to reconsider and re-articulate their sense of a particular experience. This can be very valuable in helping them to sort out feelings and events.

The wide spectrum of emotion released in grief is often frightening to the bereaved. Fear, confusion, guilt, anger, and sadness emerge at unpredictable times. The result of this emotional avalanche is that the bereaved may feel overwhelmed and sapped of the energy necessary to deal with these powerful feelings. The volunteer needs to reassure the bereaved that these feelings will gradually become manageable.

The first few months of grief are more likely to be spent reviewing memories of the loved one's illness and the strain of the last few, very demanding, weeks of life. Later, the relationship itself will be reviewed—often in minute detail. Changes in the lives of the bereaved can cause them to feel suspended between two realities—the life of the past that they spent with the deceased, and the life of the present without the deceased in which they look into an uncertain, and often lonely, future. The volunteer, who is aware of this dilemma, can serve as a bridge linking the old reality with the new.

In the year that we offer follow-up services, the examination of the death and the review of the relationship with the deceased are the primary points of focus for the volunteer. At the end of a year, a questionnaire is filled out by the bereaved at the time of the volunteer's last visit. The emotional impact of the death deserves the concentrated attention of the volunteer.

Many times I demonstrate my sincere interest with an attitude of concern and an attentive silence. This time of quiet gives the bereaved enough psychological space to access some of the feelings embedded in the tragic experience of a traumatic loss. Also, I encourage the bereaved to find a balance between focusing on grief and finding relief from sadness and depression.

MAJOR STYLES OF GRIEF

My experience has taught me that there are two major grief-styles. The first is the traditional one — the one we all expect. The bereaved person cries for days, weeks or months. Gradually, the shock wears off and deep anguish follows as the permanence of the loss is realized. Although there may be minor setbacks, the journey through grief runs a predictable course. Gradually, the bereaved adjust to life without the deceased.

The second grief-style, however, runs a different course. Although these bereaved people also occupy their time finishing the business of the deceased, they seldom grieve actively. For instance, they seldom cry at my initial interview and often speak of wanting to put this difficult time behind them. Many plunge into the future. I see this style more often among the bereaved who are between 25 and 45 years old. It is not unusual for them to travel, change jobs or even remarry within the first six months. Moreover, within six to ten months after the death, a disappointment either at work or in their personal life often triggers a massive grief reaction — a result of many months of accumulated grief which can no longer be ignored. Their former flurry of activity has camouflaged the need to give vent to a host of painful feelings. By the time the volunteer intervenes, often the main symptom is panic or suicidal despair. It is important that any intervention be prompt, personal, and reassuring. If the mood does not change with the volunteer's call or visit, this is serious, and it is important to summon professional help.

CASE ILLUSTRATION

Karen was 33, attractive, energetic and outgoing. She had nursed her husband through a painful illness until his death a year and a half later. The two of them had spent their entire married life on a ranch. After her husband's death, Karen sold the livestock and put her ranch on the market. She bought a four-plex in Denver, redecorated it herself, rented some of the units, and returned to work. She saw two men casually, but her strong alliances were with her female friends. In the first five months, I met with her once and spoke with her briefly on the phone. I warned her that setbacks were possible at this vulnerable time and I left my phone number with her. Because of her many friends in the community, she needed only limited contact.

However, at the six month mark, I starting worrying about her. I called her one night and immediately felt alarmed by the flat tone of her voice. I told her that she sounded sad and asked her what was happening. She explained that her closest friend had moved away and, just 24 hours later, one of her tenants had filed a lawsuit against her. She had gone to work upset, and her co-workers had told her that she was "acting crazy" and should leave work.

We discussed how these several crises had triggered feelings of abandonment, rejection and helplessness. Our discussion of these feelings led us back to her husband's death. For the first time she spoke of their relationship, its ups and downs, and her guilt at not being able to save him from death. He had been a successful commodities broker and he was well-known for forecasting long-term trends. He was athletic and it was unthinkable to Karen that he would die in his prime. That she had been chosen to live while he was doomed to die was a puzzle to her. There is often a strongly-felt desire among the bereaved to find some rational explanation for the tragedy which now confronts them, and Karen was earnestly seeking such an answer.

I suggested that we meet soon as it was important for her to use this critical time for grieving over her multiple losses. We agreed to meet the next day. Before I hung up, I told her I wanted her to structure her time until our meeting. To plan what activities or tasks will make up the following 24 hours usually helps quell the storm of anxiety of someone overwhelmed by powerful emotions. I reminded her that she could call me at any hour during this critical time.

I met with her and discussed how she could grieve more fully while allowing her friends to help. We explored her relationship with her husband. She told me that they had been able to discuss his impending death, but that she had found him unreceptive to any discussion of her anguish at having to watch him die. He would get irritated with her, saying, "What are you beefing about? This isn't happening to you, it's happening to me!" She had felt squelched by him and ashamed of her feelings. I told her I wanted her to find a way to acknowledge the needs arising from her grief. I gave her a few names of therapists and I told her I would check with her soon.

In a few days I called her. I found she had taken time off from work and she had spent a day with a newly-divorced friend. They had discussed the vicissitudes of change and "starting over" for many hours. Karen was able to focus intensely on both her grief and her emotional needs for several days, and she experienced a valuable turning point. She chose not to enter therapy and gained self-esteem by mastering her personal crisis in a unique and appropriate way. She found by actively grieving a way to increase the intimacy she shared with her friends. This was invaluable in enhancing her self-esteem and in enlarging her base of support. In the ensuing months I saw her often as she confronted her grief. Karen was motivated to overcome her inhibitions about grieving. This commitment renewed her spirit and brought her a new appreciation of her many strengths which included perseverance and courage.

DISCUSSION

I learned from Karen that every individual needs to find a unique and personal solution to each crisis. With emotional support and encouragement most people have this potential. It seems that this second style of grief has a prolonged initial stage of shock or denial. The next stage of protest is intense and marked by significant activity and progress. If triggered by crisis, the bereaved person is highly motivated to find a resolution and is very open to intervention. For those who wish to explore personal issues in depth, therapy can be very useful. Our Hospice offers support groups for the bereaved to give them a community where they feel they can belong. Sometimes, the bereaved need additional assistance. For those who get stuck in grief and do not feel they are progressing, therapy is recommended in a tactful way. To someone for whom the quality of life is greatly diminished by loss, staying alive can be an arduous task.

It takes an hour and a half for me to complete an intervention comfortably with someone in crisis. The shortest length of time I can spend and still do a good job is 45 minutes. My goals are to bring a focus to the person in crisis, to ascertain which events were significant in setting off the crisis, and to identify and support the feelings that the bereaved need to express. Then, we plan what steps to take in order to make the present situation more tolerable. The feelings that the present crisis elicits usually echo the same ones that occurred when their loved one was dying. The primary work of the volunteer is to reconnect the difficulties of the present with the loss in the past. Like Karen, the bereaved usually cannot make this connection without assistance.

I also caution the bereaved to lower their expectations concerning their own performance. This is a time to maintain, not over-achieve. The amount of energy needed to heal the inner world is great. Perhaps, an exception to this rule is hobbies — especially those connected to the arts. Fishing, painting, or piano-playing can be a source of solace. Encourage the bereaved to do as much as they desire, but, the general rule is rest. It is a good idea to avoid critical or demanding friends and relatives. Bereavement requires self-focus and lots of affection and support. Criticism only stabs at a heart already torn apart by grief.

For the first few months after the death, the bereaved examine their behavior with the loved one throughout the illness and dying process. They may ruminate over each interaction wishing they had said or done something different. This very lengthy and painful process needs to be handled with patience and sensitivity as the bereaved feel very vulnerable and demoralized during this detailed self-examination. Ironically, the more conscientious the character of the bereaved, the more critical they may be of their own performance during this stress-filled time of illness and death. Why is death so often a reproach to the living? The volunteer needs to stress the positive ways in which the bereaved aided the deceased.

The outcome of this extensive exploration is that the bereaved, out of a full expression of doubts, regrets, and other powerful feelings start to disentangle themselves from their attachment to the past, but not without much emotional turmoil. Considerable support and encouragement are needed at this time (Raphael, 1983). Because this self-scrutiny is highly personal, much trust is needed between the bereaved and the volunteer. The volunteer should take the initiative by creating an atmosphere of warmth and emotional support.

Once the loss is accepted as final, which usually takes around six to eight months, the bereaved review their entire relationship with the loved one who has died. There is a tendency to either idealize or denigrate the character of the deceased. It is important to explore carefully the logic involved in these judgments as the bereaved needs to be able to honestly assess the significance of the loss.

After this assessment, the bereaved is more likely to begin integrating the past with the present. The joys and sorrows of the present take on more importance than those of the past. The bereaved start changing their future plans to make them more appropriate for their new situation.

As the bereaved feel more secure about living alone, they may feel that their self-sufficiency is, somehow, an insult to the memory of the deceased. For widows and widowers it may be difficult to date, have sexual relations, or live independently without guilt. The volunteer needs to inquire about these issues because guilt often plays a major role in grief. It may be that the bereaved made a promise to the deceased that needs to be discussed. It is very common for bereaved people to feel that the deceased is watching or judging them. One needs to explore any obstacle which prevents the bereaved from adjusting to the present.

A focus on the assets and strengths of the bereaved helps to place attention on the bereaved's own potential for growth. Once a feeling of independence has been established, there may still be some uncertainty concerning the future. As one young widow said, "I don't feel like a widow anymore, but I don't know how to be single."

It is difficult for those in grief to learn to tailor plans to suit their own needs. The volunteer needs to help the bereaved to:

1. look at their unique tastes and desires.
2. feel comfortable about trying new behaviors.
3. explore their own aspirations and talents.
4. establish individual goals.
5. reestablish meaningful ties with family and friends.
6. pursue creative endeavors.
7. forge new relationships and commitments.

As this process unfolds, the bereaved's new hopes become the focus of attention. The challenge is to find creative ways to carry these hopes to fulfillment.

CONCLUSION

We are all fascinated by stories of people who survive and surmount hardships and handicaps. Bereavement is one challenge none of us can avoid because loss and death are facts of life. But, we do have a choice as to how we will express and conduct ourselves in the face of adversity. We can share the pain or we can suffer privately. Given enough information and support, people are very resourceful and creative in finding authentic ways to fit tragedy into a larger context that still allows them to find meaning and richness in their own lives.

When grief is complicated by trauma, more time is needed for integration. Also, volunteers are limited in the amount of help they can realistically offer. As there are differences in background, experiences, and personality traits, not all efforts by volunteers on behalf of the bereaved will be successful. It is important to be aware that there are limitations as to how much volunteers or anyone can help someone adjust to a major loss.

Perhaps it is our fear that we are inadequate in the face of change that impedes our growth the most. Recovery from grief is facilitated by any acknowledgement of the loss, dependable support through the transition, and an appreciation of the assets and strengths the bereaved person possesses. These elements are necessary to rehabilitate anyone who suffers from physical or emotional injuries sufficient to cause a change in lifestyle or self-perception. To participate in the quest for self-rediscovery is both a difficult and an exciting adventure.

REFERENCES

Bowlby, John (1980). *Loss: Sadness and Depression*. New York: Basic Books, Inc.

Parkes, Colin Murray (1972). *Bereavement: Studies of Grief in Adult Life*. New York: International Universitities Press, Inc.

Raphael, Beverley (1983). *The Anatomy of Bereavement*. New York: Basic Books, Inc.